Managing Challenging Behaviour Following Acquired Brain Injury

This empirically based book provides conceptual knowledge and practical advice to enable clinicians to implement evidence-based methods drawn from learning theory for managing the catastrophic effects of challenging behaviour as an enduring outcome of acquired brain injury (ABI).

Based on a conceptual framework of neurobehavioural disability, the book takes a holistic case formulation approach, incorporating functional assessment procedures arising from the operant learning tradition that underpins the design of treatment interventions. It bridges the knowledge gap in uniquely providing a single resource to enable practitioners to implement evidence-based methods to better manage ABI behaviour disorders. The authors, who are leading experts in the field, have described a model of intervention based on a functional analytic approach to understanding behaviour within an operant learning framework. The chapters provide a step-by-step approach to assessment, formulation, intervention and evaluation of behaviour support plans, and feature examples for specific challenging behaviours in a variety of different contexts. The book is organised to support the use of this model through expert contributions concerning the origins of challenging behaviour, assessment methods and formulation, and interventions.

The practical orientation of this book makes it an indispensable read for neuropsychologists, clinical psychologists and other rehabilitation specialists involved in the care of people with ABI as well as researchers in these fields.

Nick Alderman is Senior Clinical Director, Head of Psychology and Consultant Clinical Neuropsychologist at Elysium Neurological Services, Elysium Healthcare, UK, and Honorary Professor at Swansea University, UK. He is acknowledged as an expert in neurobehavioural rehabilitation, having accrued over four decades' experience in this field. He has combined successful careers in both clinical and academic psychology, and has a proven track record in treatment innovation, service development, leadership, research and teaching. Research interests include the role of executive function impairment in challenging behaviour and the development of bespoke outcome and other measurement instruments for use in neurorehabilitation.

Andrew Worthington is Honorary Professor in the Faculty of Medicine, Health and Life Sciences at Swansea University and has been a Consultant Clinical Neuropsychologist for over 30 years. He is the director of Headwise, an independent practice for children and adults with brain injury, and is an expert in neurorehabilitation. He has lectured and published widely in the field across a range of neuropsychological conditions and has a particular clinical interest in the management of executive and behaviour disorders.

Neuropsychological Rehabilitation: A Modular Handbook

Neuropsychological rehabilitation is influenced by a number of fields both from within and outside psychology. Neuropsychology, behavioural psychology and cognitive psychology have each played important roles in the development of current rehabilitation practice, along with findings from studies of neuroplasticity, linguistics, geriatric medicine, neurology and other fields. *Neuropsychological Rehabilitation: A Modular Handbook* series reflects the broad theoretical base of the discipline, and is not confined to one conceptual framework. Although each volume is based on a strong theoretical foundation relevant to the topic in question, the main thrust of the majority of the books is the development of practical, clinical methods of rehabilitation arising out of this research enterprise.

The series is aimed at neuropsychologists, clinical psychologists and other rehabilitation specialists such as occupational therapists, speech and language pathologists, rehabilitation physicians and other disciplines involved in the rehabilitation of people with brain injury.

Series Editors: Barbara A. Wilson and Ian Robertson

For more information about this series, please visit: https://www.routledge.com/Neuropsychological-Rehabilitation-A-Modular-Handbook/book-series/SE0515

Managing Challenging Behaviour Following Acquired Brain Injury

Assessment, Intervention and Measuring Outcomes

Edited by Nick Alderman and Andrew Worthington

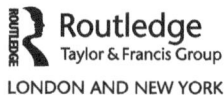

Routledge
Taylor & Francis Group

LONDON AND NEW YORK

Designed cover image: Getty Images

First published 2024
by Routledge
4 Park Square, Milton Park, Abingdon, Oxon OX14 4RN

and by Routledge
605 Third Avenue, New York, NY 10158

Routledge is an imprint of the Taylor & Francis Group, an informa business

British Library Cataloguing-in-Publication Data
A catalogue record for this book is available from the British Library

ISBN: 978-0-367-53773-9 (hbk)
ISBN: 978-0-367-53772-2 (pbk)
ISBN: 978-1-003-08329-0 (ebk)

DOI: 10.4324/9781003083290

Typeset in Times New Roman
by SPi Technologies India Pvt Ltd (Straive)

Contents

SECTION III
Intervention   93

Figures

Tables and Boxes

Abbreviations

A&E	accident and emergency
ABA	applied behaviour analysis
ABC	Antecedent–Behaviour–Consequences
ABI	acquired brain injury
ABS	Agitated Behaviour Scale
AI	artificial intelligence
BIM	best interests meeting
CBT	cognitive behavioural therapy
CHC	Continuing Healthcare
CPA	care programme approach
CQC	Care Quality Commission
CSW	clinical support worker
CT	computerised tomography
DHT	digital health technology
DoLS	Deprivation of Liberty Safeguards
DRI	differential reinforcement of incompatible behaviour
DRL	differential reinforcement of low rates of behaviour
DRO	differential reinforcement of other behaviour
EDS	episodic dyscontrol syndrome
EFAn	experimental functional analysis
EPS	Emotional Problems Scale
FA	functional assessment
FAM	Female Additional Manual
FAn	functional analysis
FBA	functional behaviour assessment
FND	functional neurological disorder
GAS	Goal Attainment Scale
GLM	Good Lives Model
HCR-20	Historical Clinical Risk-20
IDT	interdisciplinary team
ISB	inappropriate sexual behaviour
MCA	Mental Capacity Act (2005)
MDT	multidisciplinary team

MHA	Mental Health Act (1983)
MTC	major trauma centre
NBD	neurobehavioural disability
NbR	neurobehavioural rehabilitation
NCR	non-contingent reinforcement
NEAD	non-epileptic attack disorder
NG	nasogastric
NHS	National health Service
NICE	National Institute for Clinical Excellence
OAS	Overt Aggression Scale
OAS-MNR	Overt Aggression Scale – Modified for Neurorehabilitation
OBS	Overt Behaviour Scale
ORM	observational recording measures
PBS	positive behaviour support
PBS+PLUS	Positive Behaviour Support + Plus
PEG	percutaneous endoscopic gastrostomy
PERMA	Positive Emotion, Engagement, Relationships, Meaning, and Accomplishments
PTA	post-traumatic amnesia
PTMF	Power Threat Meaning Framework
PTSD	post-traumatic stress disorder
RCT	randomised controlled trial
RSVP	Risk of Sexual Violence Protocol
RTC	road traffic collision
SAH	subarachnoid haemorrhage
SALT	speech and language therapy
SASBA	St Andrew's Sexual Behaviour Assessment
SASNOS	St Andrew's–Swansea Neurobehavioural Outcomes Scale
SCED	single case experimental design
SMT	self-monitoring training
SPJ	structured professional judgement
START	Short-Term Assessment of Risk and Treatability
SVR-20	Sexual Violence Risk-20
TBI	traumatic brain injury
TDT	transdisciplinary team
TOOTS	time-out-on-the-spot
UNCRPD	United Nations Convention on the Rights of Persons with Disabilities
VRAG	Violence Risk Appraisal Guide
WPTA	Westmead post-traumatic amnesia

Contributors

Nick Alderman is Senior Clinical Director, Head of Psychology and Consultant Clinical Neuropsychologist at Elysium Neurological Services, Elysium Healthcare, UK, and Honorary Professor at Swansea University, UK.

Jenny Brooks is a Consultant Clinical Psychologist working in independent practice in the UK.

Niall Diggin is Safe and Therapeutic Management of Aggression and Violence Regional Lead at Elysium Neurological Services, Elysium Healthcare, UK.

Clark Gilkes is a Consultant Clinical Case Manager working as an associate at Karen Burgin Ltd, UK, and Managing Director of Three Pillars Rehabilitation, UK.

Caroline Knight is a Consultant Clinical Neuropsychologist and Head of Psychology and Therapeutic Programme working in brain injury rehabilitation at The Oakleaf Group, UK, and Honorary Lecturer at the University of Leicester, UK.

Abigail Methley is a Clinical Psychologist in independent practice and an Honorary Associate with the Open University, UK

Paul Mooney is Clinical Director for Service Development and Improvement at Elysium Neurological Services, Elysium Healthcare, UK, Honorary Assistant Professor at the School of Medicine, University of Nottingham, UK, and Visiting Fellow at the School of Psychology, University of Lincoln, UK.

Darren Smith is Lead Social Worker and Safeguarding Lead at Elysium Neurological Services, Elysium Healthcare, UK.

Alistair Teager is a Consultant Clinical Neuropsychologist at Manchester Centre for Clinical Neurosciences, UK, and has also engaged in humanitarian work for the World Health Organisation in Ukraine.

Andrew Worthington is a Consultant Clinical Neuropsychologist and Director of Headwise, an independent practice for children and adults with acquired brain injury.

Preface

Nick Alderman

What justifies me to co-edit a book on this subject? Nearly four decades have passed since completing training in clinical psychology at the University of Glasgow. In that time, I have worked almost exclusively in neurobehavioural (NbR) services; looking back, I am reminded how lucky I have been, especially in being in the right place at the right time.

It is ironic my first degree was in social psychology, in which there was no study of biological psychology, new learning or applications of operant conditioning. On graduation, I considered a career in clinical psychology, initially inspired by the experimental literature on helping the human condition. This meant entering a world of doubt and uncertainty; the number of training places was far less than the number of applicants. Seeking relevant clinical experience was a must. After a year working as a nursing assistant in an NHS psychiatric hospital in Sussex, I applied for an interesting looking job at as a therapy assistant at St Andrew's Hospital in Northampton, working in what was described as one of the 'behavioural wards'. The post carried opportunities to experience lots of low-level psychology tasks and I applied. A couple of weeks later I found myself with 15 other hopefuls in the grandeur of St Andrew's Hospital. This was my first encounter with one of the psychologists who was to have a substantial influence on my career, Rodger Wood. The interview process ran over two days, including meeting staff in the hospital social club, with the formal interview the next day. By this time, we were all enthused with wanting the job. All applicants gathered to learn from Rodger who the lucky recipient was; imagine the surprise when Rodger announced we were all going to be offered posts! A letter would follow informing us which ward would we be joining.

While waiting for my letter, I was browsing in a book shop in The Lanes in Brighton, when a volume with a distinctive green spine caught my eye. This was *Applications of Conditioning Theory*, edited by Graham Davey (1981). I randomly opened the book at a chapter written by Rodger Wood and Peter Eames, which provided a detailed account of how behaviour modification was being used to provide a unique programme to help people with acquired brain injury (ABI) with very challenging behaviour achieve their rehabilitation potential. This proved fascinating. What was more, was this unique programme was at the Kemsley Unit, St Andrew's Hospital. I purchased the book and hoped upon hope I would be picked to work there.

My letter subsequently arrived and the rest, as they say, is history. From being in the right place at the right time, and by sheer good luck, I became a member of the clinical team facilitating the very first NbR programme, with the Kemsley Unit first opening its doors to patients three years earlier in 1979. I was lucky to play a small part in the early days of this pioneering programme and to work in a clinical team organised as what we now call a transdisciplinary team, a model of working very relevant to this volume. I was especially grateful for the opportunity of working with the early pioneers of NbR, including Professor Rodger Wood, Dr Peter Eames, Ian Fussey, Keith Hawley, Bob Merriman and Jakki Livesey-van Dorst.

Serendipity was responsible for me meeting many of my key influencers. I must mention Professor Paul Burgess. I met Paul when I returned to the Kemsley Unit, where we developed some innovative behavioural interventions. Paul moved to progress his academic career at University College London with Professor Tim Shallice. I was keen to develop a research role integral to my clinical career, and I liked the idea of publishing but had little confidence with this. Paul invited me to collaborate on a couple of book chapters, drawing from clinical cases we had worked on, to demonstrate how the theories of frontal lobe function he was developing explained both the origins of challenging behaviour and how operant learning interventions helped remediate these (Burgess and Alderman, 1990; Alderman and Burgess, 1990). An important aspect of Paul's pioneering work explained the discrepancies sometimes found between normal test performance vs impaired functioning in the real world, resulting in the Six Elements Test and Multiple Errands Test (Shallice and Burgess, 1991). This led to further collaboration on several related projects (e.g., Alderman et al., 2003), including the BADS (Wilson et al., 1996).

At about the same time, as a further means of developing a parallel career in research, I was hunting for a PhD supervisor. Continuing the theme of being in the right place at the right time, I was assigned an assistant psychologist, Anna Wilson, daughter of Professor Barbara Wilson. Anna engineered a meeting with Barbara who very kindly agreed to be my supervisor. I combined research with my clinical work, the theme being further extension of my work with Paul. A minority of patients admitted to the Kemsley Unit proved unresponsive; my PhD was concerned with determining reasons for this and developing new ways of working. During this time Barbara was appointed at what was then the MRC Applied Psychology Unit, and supervision sessions moved to Cambridge. This gave me further opportunities, including participation in the weekly seminars, and also the privilege of meeting some very notable psychologists, including Professor Ian Robertson and Professor Alan Baddeley, both of who were kind enough to take an interest in my research. Following the success of the Rivermead Behavioural Memory Test (Wilson, Cockburn and

Baddeley, 1985), Barbara wanted to develop a similar measure that circumvented many of the reasons underpinning mixed validity of existing measures of executive functioning using tests that were analogues of everyday tasks. Paul became a founding member of this project. We were subsequently joined by Jon Evans and Hazel Emslie, a successful collaboration that created the Behavioural Assessment of the Dysexecutive Syndrome (BADS) (Wilson et al., 1996), the pilot version of which was a chapter in my PhD.

My third key influencer has already been mentioned. Professor Rodger Wood left the Kemsley Unit shortly after my return from clinical psychology training, moving on to help create what would become the Brain Injury Rehabilitation Trust (BIRT). I have had the good fortune to continue to collaborate with Rodger. He returned to Wales to a post at Swansea University, and, as a consequence, I have held honorary positions there for the last 20 years. Together with my good friend and colleague Dr Claire Williams at Swansea, the three of us continue to work on various projects, most notably the St Andrew's–Swansea Neurobehavioural Outcomes Scale (SASNOS) (Alderman, Wood and Williams, 2011), exploration of its psychometric properties (e.g., Alderman et al., 2017), its application (e.g., Alderman, Williams and Wood, 2021) and further development of the instrument (Alderman, Williams and Wood, 2018). Our small group at Swansea has further benefitted from Andrew Worthington joining through his appointment at the university (Williams et al., 2020).

The net effect of my key influencers and experience over four decades has enabled me to develop new approaches within NbR. However, this was only possible because of the earlier research regarding use of behavioural interventions pioneered by Rodger Wood, Peter Eames and others at the Kemsley Unit. This bought together a range of theoretical frameworks, including neuropsychology, that, for the first time, enabled understanding not only of how new learning is restrained by cognitive impairment, but also of how this underpins challenging behaviour. If this information is not considered in the formulation and the design of behaviour support plans, they are unlikely to be effective. When lecturing on the subject, Rodger makes the point that clinicians need to properly understand brain function and the role the damaged brain plays in disability; without this, rehabilitation interventions will fail, and I fully agree with him. Referrals to NbR services are usually pre-dated by multi-page positive behaviour support (PBS) plans that have not succeeded because these points have not been considered (see Chapter 7).

My own interests include the relationship between executive functioning impairment and challenging behaviour, in particular, how poor self-monitoring underpins evolution of these behaviours, and development of approaches to reduce behaviour disturbance secondary to it (e.g., Alderman, Fry and Youngson, 1995). I have also been struck by the paucity of assessment and measurement instruments developed specifically for neurorehabilitation and have strived to help fill some of these gaps. In addition to the SASNOS, further examples of this aspect of my work include two observational recording measures frequently referenced throughout this volume, the Overt Aggression Scale – Modified for Neurorehabilitation (OAS-MNR) (Alderman, Knight and Morgan, 1997 and the St Andrew's Sexual Behaviour Assessment (SASBA) (Knight et al., 2008).

There is insufficient provision of NbR services in the UK, a consequence of lack of awareness about ABI and its consequences. Many survivors never receive specialist rehabilitation; and many gravitate to services for containment purposes because of challenging behaviour (see Chapter 1). This book is written by clinicians to assist clinicians working with these people, offering a model to guide intervention (Chapter 2), a range of techniques to utilise (Chapter 6) and practical advice regarding both the context within which this is made, and categories of challenging behaviour typically encountered. Contributing authors are all clinicians who are experts in their field, and I hope the content offered will go some way to ensuring more people with ABI achieve better outcomes.

Andrew Worthington

I have been extremely fortunate to work alongside a number of inspirational and leading figures in neuropsychology and neuropsychiatry from an early stage of my career. It is difficult to recognise the influence of one's colleagues at the time, but given the opportunity this book presents to reflect on how my interest in neurobehavioural rehabilitation developed and my own contribution, it seemed to me that the wheels were set in motion much earlier than I had previously considered.

My interest in the brain and particularly the frontal lobe began at school with a fortuitous acquisition of Luria's 1973 popular volume *The Working Brain* as my choice for a school Scripture prize. This was cemented at university when, thanks to my undergraduate mentor Graham Powell, I spent a year at the Maudsley Hospital in south London during which time I was fortunate to attend both neuropathology seminars with the renowned Professor Peter Lantos and clinical ward rounds with Professor Alwyn Lishman, author of the seminal textbook *Organic Psychiatry*. Professor of experimental psychopathology, Isaac Marks, had just published his *Fears, Phobias and Rituals* (Marks, 1987), which expounded the behavioural basis for treatment of a range of anxiety disorders. There can be no better training than early exposure to the complexity of brain and behaviour relations within a stimulating clinical-academic environment where skilled observation and assessment mixed with rigorous analytical thinking, combines with compassion and sensitivity.

On returning to the Maudsley Hospital to complete my clinical training at the Institute of Psychiatry (as it was then called), my first and final placements were in neuropsychology with Dr Maria Wyke and Professor Tom McMillan and they provided a firm foundation for neuropsychological assessment and rehabilitation respectively. The department of psychology was formerly headed by Hans Eysenck, who had been a strong advocate of behavioural interventions for mental health problems. By the time of my training Professor Jeffrey

Gray was head of department, and his work on animal learning, including blocking and latent inhibition in schizophrenia, his notion of reinforcement sensitivity, and his short biography of Pavlov (Gray, 1979) provided an important grounding in learning theory. It was thanks to Graham Powell again whose short but bold book *Brain and Personality* (Powell, 1979) integrating the conditioning theories of Eysenck and Gray with the effects of brain injury, showed me a way of combining behavioural principles with neuropsychology.

It was my subsequent clinical work at Grafton Manor, under the inspired leadership of Dr Peter Eames, that introduced me to neurobehavioural rehabilitation in practice and there is no better description of how to build an effective transdisciplinary team than the experience encapsulated by Eames, Turnbull and Goodman-Smith (1989). Yet, having previously completed the Institute of Neurology course in clinical cognitive neuropsychology, the lack of a cognitive aspect to a rigidly behavioural regime was ultimately unsatisfying. My clinical training had brought me into contact with Paul Burgess, then undertaking his PhD with Professor Tim Shallice at University College London, from which the Hayling and Brixton tests were to emerge. I was impressed by the application of neuropsychological theory to better understand behaviour disorder – illustrated by Shallice and Burgess (1991) on strategy application disorder, introducing the world to the Six Elements and Multiple Errands tests – and the potential for theoretically informed intervention (reflected in Burgess and Alderman, 1990). This led to my own PhD with Professor Shallice on the topic of disorders of temporal experience in severe brain injury and my reformulation of strategy application disorder as a planning deficit associated with autobiographical memory impairment (Worthington, 1999) rather than a selective prospective memory disorder as others had proposed (Burgess and Shallice, 1997). This then led to further work on the amelioration of executive deficits underlying behaviour disorder (Worthington, 2003a; Worthington and Archer, 2009; Worthington and Waller, 2009; Wood and Worthington, 2017).

The 1990s was a fruitful time for neuropsychology and I began a clinical collaboration with Professor Rodger Wood at the Brain Injury Rehabilitation Trust (Wood and Worthington, 1999, 2001a, 2001b; Worthington and Wood, 2008) and, by the end of that decade, I had the opportunity to establish a new residential community service for adults with challenging behaviour (Worthington, 2003b). Over time, exposed to daily financial imperatives to secure funding and demonstrate value for money for neurobehavioural services, I developed an interest in commissioning and health economics, which led to further postgraduate study and research on cost-effectiveness (Worthington and Oldham, 2006; Worthington et al., 2006) and how efficiency should be an important consideration alongside effectiveness in neuropsychological rehabilitation more generally (Worthington, da Silva Ramos and Oddy, 2017).

Looking back, much has changed but the clinical challenges remain the same. Certain aspects that have always been central to neurobehavioural services, such as non-medical leadership, transdisciplinary work and joint goal setting, are now found in other types of service. The background to professional practice has evolved, as reviewed by Darren Smith and me in Chapter 3. Clinicians should be aware of the history of their discipline (see Worthington, Wood and McMillan, 2016) and not lose sight of the practical benefit of a good theory. It is satisfying to observe the integration of cognitive and behavioural constructs applied on a daily basis to neurobehavioural rehabilitation and the potential for new technologies (Worthington, 2016, 2017). Services are being developed for a range of complex conditions with behaviours that challenge, and it is gratifying to see functional neurological disorders come in from the cold.

This is a clinical book, reflecting the dedication, wisdom and experience of a number of skilled clinicians, not only the authors to whom the editors are especially grateful but also the many people whose work has inspired and encouraged the current generation of practitioners to ply their trade in this fascinating and rewarding field. We hope that this book will prove of practical benefit to psychologists and others working with challenging behaviour in its many guises and that it may encourage others to embrace the opportunity to do so.

References

Alderman, N. and Burgess, P.W. (1990). Integrating cognition and behaviour: A pragmatic approach to brain-injury rehabilitation. In R.Ll. Wood and I. Fussey (eds), *Cognitive Rehabilitation in Perspective*. Abingdon: Taylor & Francis Ltd.

Alderman, N., Burgess, P.W., Knight, C. and Henman, C. (2003). Ecological validity of a simplified version of the Multiple Errands Test. *Journal of the International Neuropsychological Society*, *9*, 31–44.

Alderman, N., Fry, R.K. and Youngson, H.A. (1995). Improvement of self-monitoring skills, reduction of behaviour disturbance and the dysexecutive syndrome: Comparison of response cost and a new programme of self-monitoring training. *Neuropsychological Rehabilitation*, *5*, 193–221.

Alderman, N., Knight, C. and Morgan, C. (1997). Use of a modified version of the Overt Aggression Scale in the measurement and assessment of aggressive behaviours following brain injury. *Brain Injury*, *11*, 503–523.

Alderman, N., Williams, C., Knight, C. and Wood, R.Ll. (2017). Measuring change in symptoms of neurobehavioural disability: Responsiveness of the St Andrew's–Swansea Neurobehavioural Outcomes Scale (SASNOS). *Archives of Clinical Neuropsychology*, *32* (8), 951–962.

Alderman, N., Williams, C. and Wood, R.Ll. (2018). When normal scores don't equate to independence: Recalibrating ratings of neurobehavioural disability from the 'St Andrew's–Swansea Neurobehavioural Outcome Scale' to reflect context-dependent support. *Brain Injury*, *32* (2), 218–229.

Alderman, N., Williams, C. and Wood, R.Ll. (2021). Using the St Andrew's–Swansea Neurobehavioural Outcome Scale (SASNOS) to determine prevalence and predictors of neurobehavioural disability amongst survivors with traumatic brain injury in the community. *Neuropsychological Rehabilitation*, *32* (9), 2342–2369.

Alderman, N., Wood, R.Ll. and Williams, C. (2011). The development of the St Andrew's–Swansea Neurobehavioural Outcome Scale: Validity and reliability of a new measure of neurobehavioural disability and social handicap. *Brain Injury*, *25*, 83–100.

Burgess, P.W. and Alderman, N. (1990). Rehabilitation of dyscontrol syndromes following frontal lobe damage: A cognitive neuropsychological approach. In R.Ll. Wood and I. Fussey (eds), *Cognitive Rehabilitation in Perspective*. Abingdon: Taylor & Francis, 183–203.

Burgess, P.W. and Shallice, T. (1997.) The relationship between prospective and retrospective memory: Neuropsychological evidence. In M.A. Conway (ed.), *Cognitive Models of Memory* (pp. 247–272). Hove: Taylor and Francis.

Davey, G. (ed.) (1981). *Applications of Conditioning Theory*. London: Methuen & Co.

Eames, P., Turnbull, J. and Goodman-Smith, A. (1989) Service delivery and assessment of program. In D. Lezak (ed.), *Assessment of the Behavioral Consequences of Head Trauma* (pp. 195–214). New York: Alan Liss.

Gray, J.A. (1979). *Pavlov*. London: Fontana.

Knight, C., Alderman, N., Johnson, C., Green, S., Birkett-Swan, L. and Yorston, G. (2008). The St Andrew's Sexual Behaviour Assessment (SASBA): Development of a standardised recording instrument for the measurement and assessment of challenging sexual behaviour in people with progressive and acquired neurological impairment. *Neuropsychological Rehabilitation*, *18*, 129–159.

Luria, A.R. (1973) *The Working Brain*. Harmondsworth: Penguin Books.

Marks, I. (1987). *Fears, Phobias and Rituals. Panic, Anxiety and their Disorders*. Oxford: Oxford University Press.

Powell, G.E. (1979). *Brain and Personality*. Farnborough: Saxon House.

Shallice, T. and Burgess, P.W. (1991). Deficits in strategy application following frontal lobe damage in man. *Brain*, *114* (2), 727–741.

Williams, C., Wood, R.Ll., Alderman, N. and Worthington, A. (2020). The psychosocial impact of neurobehavioural disability. *Frontiers in Neurology*, *11*, 119.

Wilson, B.A., Alderman, N., Burgess, P.W., Emslie, H. and Evans, J.J. (1996). *Behavioural Assessment of the Dysexecutive Syndrome*. Bury St Edmunds: Thames Valley Test Company.

Wilson, B.A., Cockburn, J. and Baddeley, A.D. (1985). *The Rivermead Behavioural Memory Test*. Bury St Edmunds: Thames Valley Test Company.

Wood, R.Ll. and Eames, P. (1981). Application of behaviour modification in the treatment of traumatically brain-injured adults. In G. Davey (ed.), *Applications of Conditioning Theory* (pp. 81–101). London: Methuen & Co.

Wood, R.Ll. and Worthington, A.D. (1999). Outcome in community rehabilitation: Measuring the social impact of disability. *Neuropsychological rehabilitation*, *9* (3–4), 505–516.

Wood, R.Ll. and Worthington, A. (2001a). Neurobehavioural rehabilitation: A conceptual paradigm. In R.Ll. Wood and T.M. McMillan (eds), *Neurobehavioural Disability and Social Handicap Following Traumatic Brain Injury* (pp. 107–131). Hove: Psychology Press.

Wood, R.Ll. and Worthington, A. (2001b). Neurobehavioural rehabilitation in practice. In R.Ll. Wood and T.M. McMillan (eds), *Neurobehavioural Disability and Social Handicap Following Traumatic Brain Injury* (pp. 133–155). Hove: Psychology Press.

Wood, R.Ll. and Worthington, A. (2017). Neurobehavioural abnormalities associated executive dysfunction after traumatic brain injury. *Frontiers in Behavioral Neuroscience*. http://doi.org/10.3389/fnbeh.2017.00195

Worthington, A. (1999). Dysexecutive paramnesia: Strategic retrieval deficits in retrospective and prospective remembering. *Neurocase*, *5* (1), 47–57.

Worthington, A. (2003a). The natural recovery and treatment of executive disorders. In P.W. Halligan, U. Kischka and J.C. Marshall (eds), *Handbook of Clinical Neuropsychology*. New York: Oxford University Press.

Worthington, A (2003b). Out on a limb? Developing an integrated rehabilitation service for adults with acquired brain injury. *Clinical Psychology*, *23*, 14–18.

Worthington, A. (2016). Treatments and technologies in the rehabilitation of apraxia and action disorganisation syndrome. *Journal of Neurorehabilitation*, *39*, 163–174.

Worthington, A. (2017). Emerging technologies for the rehabilitation of executive dysfunction and action disorganisation. *Austin Journal of Clinical Neurology*, *4* (4), 1116.

Worthington, A. and Archer, N. (2009). Assessment and management of risk. In M. Oddy and A. Worthington (eds), *Rehabilitation of Executive Disorders Following Brain Injury* (pp. 299–326). Oxford: Oxford University Press.

Worthington, A., da Silva Ramos, S. and Oddy, M. (2017). The cost effectiveness of neuropsychological rehabilitation. In B. Wilson, J. Winegardner, C.M. Van Heughten and T. Ownsworth (eds), *International Handbook of Neuropsychological Rehabilitation* (pp. 469–479). Abingdon: Routledge.

Worthington, A.D., Matthews, S., Melia, Y. and Oddy, M. (2006). Cost-benefits associated with social outcome from neurobehavioural rehabilitation. *Brain Injury*, *20* (9), 947–957.

Worthington, A. and Oldham, J.B. (2006). Delayed discharge from rehabilitation after brain injury. *Clinical Rehabilitation*, *20*, 79–82.

Worthington, A. and Waller, J. (2009). Rehabilitation of activities of daily living. In M. Oddy and A. Worthington (eds), *Rehabilitation of Executive Disorders Following Brain Injury* (pp. 195–210). Oxford: Oxford University Press.

Worthington, A. and Wood, R.Ll. (2008). Behaviour problems. In A. Tyerman and N. King (eds), *Psychological Approaches to Rehabilitation After Traumatic Brain Injury* (pp. 227–259). Oxford: Blackwell.

Worthington, A., Wood, R.Ll. and McMillan, T.M. (2016). Perspective on neurobehavioural disability over the past four decades. In R.Ll. Wood and T.M. McMillan (eds), *Neurobehavioural Disability and Social Handicap After Traumatic Brain Injury*. Hove: Psychology Press.

Section I
Origins of challenging behaviour

1 Outcomes from acquired brain injury

Prevalence and impact of challenging behaviour

Nick Alderman and Andrew Worthington

What is an acquired brain injury?

Acquired brain injury is an injury of sudden onset that occurs after birth and is not a consequence of a genetic or congenital disorder. Causes include lack of oxygen to the brain (hypoxia), stroke, haemorrhage, cerebral tumours, exposure to toxins, and infections such as encephalitis or meningitis.

Traumatic brain injury (TBI) is one form of ABI that is particularly prevalent in services that manage challenging behaviour by virtue of the fronto-temporal emphasis of many brain traumas, whether the brain is exposed (open) or the skull remains intact (closed). In the latter case, injury is a consequence of mechanical forces operating on the brain due to rapid changes in velocity such as occurs in high-speed road traffic accidents, and of compression (from swelling of brain tissue following trauma or from accumulation of blood within the cranial cavity).

What outcomes are associated with ABI?

Survivors of ABI comprise a heterogeneous population with a wide variety of needs, encompassing physical, functional, cognitive, emotional, behavioural and psychosocial changes. With regard to TBI, younger people tend to make a better recovery, but only about 15 per cent of 'severe' cases return to employment within five years (Winslade, 1999). However, there remains a general lack of awareness about ABI and its consequences among the general public and healthcare workers, including medical practitioners. As a condition ABI is poorly understood. Survivors may acquire life-changing disabilities but still appear 'normal' except to those who know them well. Reviews confirm ABI constitutes a chronic condition with 'hidden' disabilities, often referred to as a 'silent epidemic'.

More people survive because of advances in acute medical care. In the UK, ABI impacts on around 8.5 per cent of the population, with TBI being most prevalent. While most are categorised as mild, effects of ABI can be catastrophic and pervasive. In the UK, a report prepared by the All-Party Parliamentary Group on ABI (2018) collated a range of statistics that described the

DOI: 10.4324/9781003083290-2

problem. It was found there has been a 10 per cent increase in hospital admissions of people presenting with ABI, amounting to 900,000 annually. Consequently, the number of survivors living with chronic disabilities is huge. The prevalence of TBI is estimated at 1.3 million, inflicting costs in excess of 17 billion euros, equivalent to 10 per cent of the UK's National Health Service budget.

Whilst outcomes are variable, long-term neurocognitive impairment is very characteristic, especially in TBI. Impaired consciousness and post-traumatic amnesia (PTA) are hallmarks of this condition, but typically are resolved within hours or days. However, persistent, severe neurocognitive deficits are associated with moderate and severe TBI, with as many as 65 per cent of survivors reporting long-term problems compared to 15 per cent of those classified with mild TBI. A broad range of difficulties is experienced, including deficits in attention and memory, processing speed, awareness, executive functions, communication, visuospatial abilities and general intelligence (see Rabinowitz and Levin, 2014, for a detailed account of cognitive sequelae of TBI).

Chronic neurocognitive impairment contributes to the 'hidden' disabilities associated with ABI, often described as a 'silent epidemic' of ABI because their presence is not obvious from casual observation. The presence of physical and sensory disabilities due to problems such as paresis, ataxia, visual impairment, imbalance and poor mobility can exacerbate the neurobehavioural sequelae and complicate rehabilitation.

Whilst the physical consequences of ABI are frequently apparent on initial observation, a more intimate acquaintance over a longer period by multiple informants may be necessary to appreciate the full extent of the emotional and psychosocial disorders that can persist after severe ABI. A substantial literature review by Stéfan and colleagues (Stéfan, Mathé and SOFMER group, 2016) revealed that many studies, including those investigating outcomes years after injury, found evidence of mood disorders, including depression (12–76 per cent), anxiety (0.8–24.5 per cent) and obsessive-compulsive disorders (1.2–30 per cent). Agitation was a frequent characteristic of TBI with an average incidence of 46 per cent. Rates of irritability ranged from 29 to 71 per cent. Apathy (loss of goal-directed behaviours) mirrored these findings, with prevalence rates varying between 20 and 71 per cent.

Challenging behaviour as a consequence of ABI

Relatives and professionals often refer to people suffering personality change after brain injury when the underlying concern is that a person's behaviour has changed, usually for the worse. The presence of significant behaviour change is acknowledged as posing a greater impediment to community integration in survivors of TBI than physical disabilities (Baguley, Cooper and Felmingham, 2006; Tateno, Jage and Robinson, 2003).

Challenging behaviour has potentially catastrophic consequences and its presence has been associated with a variety of undesirable outcomes, including chronic difficulties with interpersonal relationships, marital breakdown and family disintegration, failure to return to work, increased risk of psychiatric disorder and offending behaviour. Challenging behaviour as a legacy of ABI is frequently enduring. Increased risk to self and others can result in exclusion from mainstream neurorehabilitation, with survivors being discharged home without exploring their potential for recovery and without appropriate levels of support. Families and communities unable to cope may also exclude survivors, resulting in homelessness or, ultimately, survivors being placed with services purely for management purposes such as care homes and psychiatric hospitals, rather than being provided with appropriate rehabilitation.

The situation is compounded by a lack of awareness about ABI and its consequences. For example, people with ABI who have infringed laws are often dealt with by imprisonment or admission to secure forensic psychiatric services. People with ABI are over-represented among offender populations; surveys typically suggest 50 per cent or more of prison inmates have sustained at least one TBI compared with 12 per cent in the general population, typically offending at a younger age and more frequently than neurologically healthy prisoners. It should be no surprise that increased recidivism rates among offenders with ABI compared to those with no history of injury, further suggest that custodial sentences do not constitute effective rehabilitation (Williams, 2012).

What challenging behaviours are a legacy of ABI?

Given their potentially catastrophic impact, what form does behaviour change take? A good starting point is the description by Broe et al. (1981), which captures well the nature of the sudden and unexpected alteration in the conduct of people who sustain a brain injury:

> such patients may be impulsive, emotionally labile, disinhibited, aggressive, and as a consequence of their impairment have lost insight into their emotional response. So while physically and cognitively well recovered ... [these] patients experience deficits which have adverse effects on their interpersonal relationships and return to employment.
>
> (Walsh, 1985, p. 145)

There is acknowledgement that the diversity of behaviour change and challenges it imposes is considerable, ranging from difficulties in initiating basic activities, to property destruction and physical assaults. Whilst these represent two ends of an extreme, both increase risk to the survivors and others. As odd as it may seem, given the consequences of behaviour change for the survivor, their family and community, there is surprisingly little consideration about what constitutes 'challenging behaviour'. We advocate two perspectives that should be consulted. The first is behaviour change and challenging behaviour as it is described within the literature; the second, behaviours considered challenging within the clinical context.

Challenging behaviour – the literature

There is no universal taxonomy of behaviour change associated with ABI, and within the literature there is considerable variation regarding type and extent of behaviour change. Furthermore, there is lack of consensus in defining thresholds to be crossed in order for behaviour to be regarded as sufficiently challenging to require intervention. Many accounts describe behaviours that would be considered examples of 'positive' behaviour disorders, that is, conduct initiated by an individual as undesirable, including aggression and sexually inappropriate behaviour. At the other end of the spectrum is the absence of purposeful behaviour, where an individual fails to initiate skilled actions, for example bathing, washing and changing clothes, resulting in personal neglect. In the midst of this range lies a wide spectrum of idiosyncratic behaviour changes, often described as a consequence of ABI, perceived as symptomatic of the 'personality change' by a significant other – that the person is somehow 'not the way they used to be' before injury (Brooks et al., 1986).

It is perhaps for these reasons that no taxonomy, a precise definition of the total range of post-ABI behaviour disorders, is evident in the literature; and that systematic reviews of the literature regarding the extent of these changes are comparatively few (Stéfan, Mathé and SOFMER group, 2016).

Consequently, many researchers choose to focus on studying a single, readily discernible aspect of behaviour change, such as aggression. However, considerable discrepancies in incidence rates between studies is evident. For example, a review by Tateno, Jage and Robinson (2001) found incidence of aggression varied from 11 to 96 per cent. One reason for this is that there are no universally accepted definitions of what comprises the behaviours studied. The attribution of symptoms of behaviour change, for example, can lead to different classifications such as apathy and motivational disorders being interpreted as symptomatic of depression. There is also no agreement regarding their identification and measurement, with different instruments emphasising different aspects of symptoms and behaviours. Other compounding factors are differences regarding time since injury and the context, for example rehabilitation unit versus the community.

The more idiosyncratic symptoms of behaviour change are often managed by pooling them together into a more imprecise, difficult-to-measure descriptor, such as 'problems with social functioning' or 'interpersonal difficulties'. Researchers may choose to publish these as individual case studies, but sometimes they are so unique that the symptoms described are rarely observed. Frequent references in the literature to unusual, rare phenomena can lead to exaggerated estimates of their frequency in the brain injury population. Large group studies are used as the 'gold standard' in quantitative research; however, in ABI research, these can be potentially misleading too. ABI survivors collectively comprise a highly non-homogeneous population, not only in the outcomes achieved, but also regarding the causal factors underlying the presence of seemingly similar behaviour problems that are grouped together for the purposes of study. A frequent objective of larger studies is to determine causal factors through statistical analysis; this often results in disappointment, usually because the drivers of the behaviour studied can vary considerably between individuals, as we will see in other chapters in this volume.

The extent to which researchers elevate behaviour change to 'challenging behaviour' is also worthy of mention. Not all changes require attempts to 'manage' them. Some of the difficulty is attributable to a lack of consensus about what challenging behaviour is. Most behaviours described do not take place exclusively within the context of ABI; instead, they comprise a continuum, along which there is a point where it will become classed as excessive or problematic because it exceeds a threshold deemed 'normal' for the general population. Researchers using quantitative methods and psychometric measurement instruments benefit when normative data is available for neurologically healthy controls. If not, there is a risk that any 'adverse' behaviour detected is perceived as an outcome from ABI, when this is not always the case.

This has two related aspects: (i) identifying how common a particular condition is in the non-brain-injured population; and (ii) determining the normal range of behaviour. For example, from time to time everyone experiences a headache, memory lapse or irritability, so the fact that someone reports this after brain injury is not necessarily a consequence of neurological impairment. Knowing how often this occurs in the normal population (base rate information) helps to determine the likelihood of an experience being caused by the condition of interest (in our case, ABI). Yet most genuine post-brain-injury symptoms are not specific to brain injury so it is important to consider whether they can be defined in such a way to increase their discriminative power. Many people are irritable, but fewer become physically violent, and fewer still show the temporo-limbic features characteristic of episodic dyscontrol. Taking a broad definition of aggression, for example, might capture a wider range of neurobehavioural manifestations (i.e. increased sensitivity) but at the cost of being over-inclusive to normal behaviour (thereby losing specificity).

For example, Baguley, Cooper and Felmingham (2006) assessed prevalence of aggression among 228 TBI survivors up to five years after discharge from rehabilitation. At 60 months, they found that 57 per cent met criteria for aggression. However, 58 per cent of a neurologically healthy control group also met these criteria. Comparison of these figures suggests the risk of a Type I error if the finding among the TBI group had been assumed to be entirely an outcome of brain injury. This study also showed the need to consider care in how behaviours are defined; whilst overall rates of aggression were compatible, there were nevertheless differences when subtypes were considered. The two samples were found to have similar levels of verbal aggression (TBI 51 per cent vs controls 56 per cent), but prevalence of physical aggression was higher within the TBI group, including physical assaults on other people (19 per cent vs 4 per cent).

Another issue of note with the use of psychometric instruments to investigate behaviour change is the different dimensions of those behaviours captured by the measures used. In nearly all cases, frequency is reported but data concerning severity of behavioural impact is also important (Kelly et al., 2006). Describing behaviour that has severe consequences but occurs infrequently can be misleading; similarly, describing a high-frequency behaviour that has a mild impact by just how often it takes place might also exaggerate its standing relative to other more serious outcomes.

Perception of the extent of behaviour change is also influenced by the observer or rater. Poor insight and problems with awareness are often reported as a consequence of ABI, with the result that some survivors underestimate the extent of their difficulties, including behaviour. Consequently, studies that rely exclusively on self-reporting may underestimate the extent of behaviour change. Families may also adopt a broader notion of challenging behaviour than is generally accepted by clinicians and researchers. Tam et al. (2015) highlighted expression of anger, overt aggression, socially inappropriate behaviour, repetitive and dangerous behaviours, and behavioural change secondary to cognitive impairment in this regard. It was not just the immediate, adverse consequences of these behaviours that relatives found challenging, but also longer-term impact, including reduced social contact, increased stress through avoiding triggers, dropping out of education and work, reduced living standards, and changes in family dynamics and roles.

One of the important lessons from epidemiological research is that ABI (and TBI in particular) has a strong association with indices of psychosocial deprivation (Dunn, Henry and Beard, 2003). Many of the behaviours that predispose a person to suffering ABI can also be caused by brain injury. It is important, therefore, to consider the person before the injury as well as the post-injury presentation before attributing a behaviourally challenging presentation to ABI. Information about schooling, employment, relationships and forensic history may all be relevant. Even premorbid challenging behaviour, however, may have an organic or neurodevelopmental basis – many homeless people, for example, have had multiple brain injuries (Oddy et al., 2010) – and a significant brain injury may serve to exacerbate previous propensities to antisocial behaviour. Even a milder brain injury can exert disproportionate behavioural impact if superimposed on a history of previous neurological vulnerability.

There is one additional factor, which does not receive sufficient attention in the academic literature, but which is of crucial importance to clinicians. This is the need to consider how far challenging behaviour following ABI is underpinned by brain damage or can be explained in terms of reactive psychological disorder and maladaptive coping to the experience of ABI and ABI-related losses (or any unrelated life stresses). In reality, especially for more severe injuries, there is often a neurological basis, but the two are not mutually exclusive and effective management requires careful consideration of multiple contributory factors. The present volume is concerned with management of challenging behaviour that has a primary organic basis, as this is often neglected by less neurologically informed clinicians, and ultimately psychological processes are also affected by brain injury. However, clinicians should remain mindful that challenging behaviour is often multifactorial.

These studies and observations emphasise that care needs to be taken when examining the literature on outcome and not assuming that serious challenging behaviour is necessarily attributable to brain injury or by default severe enough to merit legal attention and/or clinical intervention.

All these issues can lead to bias among experts regarding the type and extent of behaviour change post-ABI and to difficulties in arriving at a balanced view regarding this aspect of outcome. Bearing these possible limitations in mind, a cross-section of some of the studies that have examined behaviour change as an outcome of ABI will be briefly considered to help give the reader a sense of the extent of not only the diversity of disorders described, but also the variability with which these are reported.

Types, longevity and impact of challenging behaviour

Whilst behaviour change is diverse, labile mood, poor impulse control, aggression and personality change are frequently described as being most characteristic (Wood, 2001). Aggression, inappropriate behaviour that causes difficulties in social situations, sexually inappropriate behaviour and repetitive behaviour, are recognised as being most problematic by ABI survivors, family members, carers and clinicians (Tam et al., 2015). Lack of initiation, a consequence of executive function impairment, reduced drive, apathy, unconcern or lack of emotional reactivity also constitute challenging behaviour (Oddy, Cattran and Wood, 2008).

Given the diversity of outcomes, drawing on some of the literature concerned with multiple, co-existing aspects of behaviour change are helpful in conveying a sense of outcome as a whole. The contribution of Kelly and colleagues (Kelly et al., 2006) has proved especially noteworthy. The authors developed a measure that captured information about the frequency, severity and impact of a range of behaviour changes considered to be challenging post-TBI. This comprised nine items, four drawn from an existing measure of aggression (as this is acknowledged to constitute a serious aspect of behaviour change), comprising verbal aggression and physical aggression against objects, self and other people. The other five items were drawn from a comprehensive review of hundreds of examples of behaviour change considered to be challenging from 543 referrals to a specialist rehabilitation service over a five-year period, namely inappropriate sexual behaviour, perseveration/repetition, wandering/absconding, inappropriate social behaviour and lack of initiation. Together, these nine items formed the Overt Behaviour Scale (OBS). Some members of this group used these items in an empirical approach to a literature search to clarify the prevalence of challenging behaviour as opposed to behaviour change (Sabaz et al., 2014). As noted above, prevalence of aggression of all types was found to vary from as low as 11 per cent to as high as 96 per cent, lack of initiation from 40.5 per cent to 71 per cent, inappropriate sexual behaviour from 6.5 per cent to 30.4 per cent, wandering/absconding from 6 per cent to 14 per cent, and perseveration in real-world contexts (as opposed to neuropsychological assessment) at 25.3%. Sabaz and colleagues were unable to determine rates for inappropriate social behaviour because it was unclear what behaviours described in the literature fell into this category. In their own study, the OBS was used to detect challenging behaviour in a large sample referred to a community brain injury rehabilitation programme. Post-injury time was variable, with 67 per cent being five years or more. Over half (267, 54 per cent) met the criteria for exhibiting one or more challenging behaviours. The most common were inappropriate social behaviour (33.3 per cent), aggression (31.9 per cent) and lack of initiation (23.1 per cent), with 35.5 per cent of the sample displaying multiple challenging behaviours.

In another large cohort study, Timmer et al. (2020) examined outcomes in 226 TBI survivors identified from a larger sample as presenting with significant behaviour disturbance six months to one year post injury. Researchers considered nine types of behavioural disturbance, including disinhibition, wandering, anger and aggression, apathy, impaired self-awareness, deficits in judgement and decision making, and impaired planning and regulation. The presence and severity of these were determined through the scrutiny of medical files and assigned a score to reflect the degree of behaviour disturbance, 'mild' vs 'serious'. The inclusion criterion for the study was a classification of at least 'mild' behaviour disturbance; but, within this group, a large proportion were further classified as presenting with 'serious' disturbance of behaviour (24 per cent). Behaviour disturbance was three times higher in survivors with a moderate or severe TBI compared to a mild TBI (35 per cent vs 13 per cent). All nine categories of behaviour disturbance were evident within both the mild and moderate/severe TBI groups. The most prevalent behaviour problems were irritation, agitation, anger and disinhibition. Anger was more prevalent among mild TBI survivors (49 per cent vs 40 per cent), whilst disinhibition was greater within the moderate/severe TBI group (55 per cent vs 33 per cent). At six months to one year post-injury, 92 per cent had returned home, despite one in four presenting with serious disturbed behaviour; those that did not return home remained resident in nursing home settings with serious behaviour disturbance. About half the sample returned to work; a main variable influencing this was presence of behaviour problems. Once home, 15 per cent experienced relational difficulties that resulted in relationships ending in 40 per cent of these cases. Timmer and colleagues noted there was a correlation between presence of behaviour disturbance and relational problems. A point to note is that, whilst a higher proportion of mild TBI survivors participated in a rehabilitation programme during the period of study (54 per cent vs 47 per cent), return to work rates were similar (60 per cent vs 61 per cent).

Difficulties with interpersonal relationships arising from the impairment of social cognition and from inappropriate behaviour are also frequently described legacies of ABI (Alderman et al., 2017). In their study of community-dwelling TBI survivors, Alderman, Williams and Wood (2021) found most participants presented with these difficulties, which took many forms. Over 70 per cent were assessed by a significant other as presenting with social interaction problems, such as not recognising when to end conversations, 64 per cent with difficulties with relationships, for example with displaying warmth and compassion, and 67 per cent in their ability to engage others successfully in social interaction, for example in being well-mannered and polite, and demonstrating interest in other people.

Studies highlight a worrying tendency for behaviour disorders to persist and aggravate over time. For example, Brooks and colleagues (1987) found 64 per cent of TBI survivors had temper control problems five years post-injury and 20 per cent exhibited increased violent behaviour. Fifteen percent of relatives reported 'threats of violence' one year post-injury, but 54 per cent reported it after five years. Johnson and Balleny (1996) found a small minority of ABI survivors had been aggressive during the acute phase of their recovery in hospital (6 per cent), but after 18 months this had greatly increased (55.5 per cent). A consistent finding is that, without rehabilitation, greater time post-injury is associated with more prevalent challenging behaviour. For example, Sabaz et al. (2014) found that 38.2 per cent of their sample met the criteria for challenging behaviour less than a year post-injury, whilst 67.1 per cent did so five years or more afterwards.

Challenging behaviour – in clinical practice

Familiarity with ABI outcomes, including types of behaviour disorder, provides an essential starting point for any clinician with a role in managing challenging behaviour. However, a different set of criteria will be deployed in the clinical context, when deciding if behaviour change is challenging to the point that merits intervention. Unlike a research context, where a single criterion or yardstick is usually employed to differentiate between behaviour change and challenging behaviour, in recognition of the multifactorial nature of challenging behaviour, multiple criteria are routinely considered in the clinical context, including formal assessment measures, structured behavioural observations, legal matters, risk of harm to self and others, views of the patient and their family, and consideration of what is lost or cannot be achieved because of the presence of such behaviour; reference will be made to these throughout this volume. However, whilst the need to decide what is challenging behaviour and a worthy rehabilitation goal may sound obvious, it is in practice often far from clear, being soaked in moral judgement and potentially an ethical minefield. The question must always be 'Is it right to try to change this person's behaviour?'. Decision making is further complicated if the person lacks capacity, which is often undermined by poor insight and serious neurocognitive impairment.

An additional factor is the views of the rehabilitation team and care staff. They will have opinions about behaviour demonstrated by people under their care, which may be by no means universally held, depending on the point at which these behaviours exceed personal thresholds held by the clinicians and carers for what they consider should be tolerated in the workplace. These too need careful management. To illustrate the lack of consensus in what clinicians consider to be challenging behaviour worthy of intervention, Alderman (2017) surveyed views from experienced clinicians working in neurorehabilitation.

First, a list of behaviours that had been recorded as being raised in clinical meetings as potential rehabilitation goals was assembled. Among the 13 items, some behaviours were objectively more likely to achieve agreement within the clinical team, including physical assaults on others and lack of cooperation in rehabilitation sessions. Others seemed more debatable, including 'being rude' and 'calling women "love"'. A separate group of clinicians were asked to rank the items in order of priority as 'challenging and requiring intervention'. Not surprisingly, the rank order showed high agreement regarding the more overt behaviours being categorised as challenging and worthy of intervention at the top of the table. However, variability in the ranking of those towards the bottom of the list still suggested perception of what constitutes challenging behaviour lacks agreement, even among rehabilitation professionals.

Making decisions regarding rehabilitation goals is not always straightforward; what a rehabilitation professional might consider important does not necessarily reflect a wider consensus. Decisions about behaviour change are perhaps the most difficult to make and are a critical stage of the intervention model described in Chapter 2 of this volume. It is essential that, as far as possible, all involved agree the goals are to be achieved. Alderman (2017) described some key factors for consideration that can assist teams in reaching a consensus.

Interpretation

Often 'snap' decisions are made regarding whether behaviour is problematic. This is partly due to different perceptions of the observer, influenced by multiple factors including beliefs, attitudes, context, local social norms, and tolerance of what is acceptable. For example, swearing in the company of friends on a night out may be conventional (even encouraged), but the same behaviour in the context of a therapy session can be interpreted as challenging behaviour.

Intent

Attributions about intent are further influenced by subjective interpretation of the observer. Observation of stressful events introduces potential bias, which can result in individuals having very different views about causation, especially those perceived as sexually motivated (Johnson, Knight and Alderman, 2006). It is essential that decision making regarding intent is conducted in a way that highlights objectivity and, by so doing, properly informs the assessment process (see Chapter 5).

Immediate impact

Determining the immediate physical, mental and emotional harm of the behaviour will further influence the likelihood that behaviour is deemed challenging (Bezeau, Bogod and Mateer, 2004) and is often the chief objective of formal risk assessment.

Long-term impact

Decision making is influenced by consideration of what impact behaviour change has on the individual's future options, including participation in rehabilitation programmes so a person can attain their optimal potential, reintegrate into family life and participate in community activities. Behaviour may be tolerated and managed in a hospital, but what about when the patient returns home? Will the family cope? The relationship between TBI and offending has already been mentioned; if left unmanaged, might the behaviour change escalate, necessitating intervention by the police and risk of imprisonment as a consequence? Evidence of increased recidivism among people with TBI managed this way clearly points to the relevance of specialised neurorehabilitation programmes as a desirable alternative.

Consideration of these factors within the context of the prevailing legislative framework further influences decisions about justifying intervention if behaviour is challenging. Deciding whether the behaviour warrants attempts at change is a complex decision involving consideration of context, risk to self and others, appreciation of what will be lost and gained by not intervening, and determining if resources to instigate change are available.

A definition of challenging behaviour

Whilst there are no universally agreed definitions of challenging behaviour, decision making regarding whether it is sufficiently serious to warrant intervention can be assisted when questions are asked regarding a useful definition. The editors of this volume have found decision making regarding elevation of behaviour change into challenging behaviour is helped by asking questions regarding not only the immediate risk inflicted on the person concerned and those around them, but also on their ability to engage in activities aimed at increasing autonomy and future opportunities that are incompatible with such behaviours. Consequently, the oft-cited definition offered by Emerson et al. (1987) regarding this issue as it applies to learning disability has relevance too for ABI in that challenging behaviour comprises conduct:

> of such an intensity, frequency or duration that the physical safety of the person or others is likely to be placed in serious jeopardy, or behaviour which is likely to seriously limit the use of, or result in the person being denied access to, ordinary community facilities.
>
> (Emerson et al., 1987, p.138)

Drawing from the above, we have found a definition of what comprises challenging behaviour in ABI is behaviour that includes conduct that a) increases the vulnerability of the person and others, b) limits or delays access to community resources, and c) constrains participation in post-acute neurorehabilitation leading to failure to exploit and attain full potential for recovery (Alderman, 2001; Alderman, 2017).

Neurobehavioural disability

Ultimately, behaviour change observed following ABI is a product of that event, but whilst there is considerable variation in the form this takes, so too are the specific variables that underpin and drive it. Correctly identifying causal factors is essential to successful managing challenging behaviour and is a central theme of this volume. To provide an effective means of managing challenging behaviour, it is important to utilise a conceptual framework that facilitates understanding of what drives these and underpins their successful management.

The concept of neurobehavioural disability (NBD) and the related intervention paradigm of neurobehavioural rehabilitation evolved for this purpose, by highlighting the underlying neurological substrate to behaviour change after ABI. These ideas originated from early approaches to understanding chronic behaviour disturbance arising from TBI inflicted in combat in the First World War, and the subsequent pioneering work of Kurt Goldstein and Alexander Luria among others in recognising the importance of the frontal lobes in the regulation of social behaviour. Their work led to succeeding clinicians and researchers further highlighting the role of the prefrontal cortex in self-regulation of behaviour. This is a frequent legacy of ABI and key to understanding many of the neuropsychological and neurobehavioural sequelae (Worthington, Wood and McMillan, 2017).

NBD highlights both neurological and neuropsychological drivers of behaviour change following ABI. Wood (2001) described NBD as comprising elements of executive and attentional dysfunction, poor insight, problems of awareness and social judgement, labile mood, poor impulse control, and personality change. Behaviour disturbance is attributed to complex interactions between damaged neural systems and neurocognitive impairment, further exacerbated by pre-environmental factors, post-injury learning and pre-morbid personality traits (Alderman, Wood and Williams, 2011).

Attempts to account for behaviour change generally distinguish between explanations with a predominantly neurological basis and those attributable to neurocognitive impairment (Wood, 2001). For example, lesions to the orbitofrontal cortex and its connections with other brain structures are especially important, being strongly linked with weakening of inhibitions (Starkstein and Robinson, 1991); while neurocognitive impairment in the form of executive function disorders resulting in lack of 'error awareness' can then result in inappropriate social behaviour (Alderman, 2003). Behaviour change that is originally a product of neurological and neurocognitive factors is then further shaped and modified by a range of other variables, of which environmental factors, post-injury learning and pre-morbid personality traits are especially relevant. Research has highlighted many other contributing factors and co-morbidities, but results are far from conclusive. For example, even the effect of severity of ABI is unclear, with some studies failing to demonstrate any association between measures of severity and challenging behaviour (e.g. Sabaz et al., 2014), whilst others suggest differences in presentation (Timmer et al., 2020). Inconsistency between findings may be partly attributable to different definitions and interpretations of both behaviour change and potential contributing factors, but they do indicate the need for individual assessment and management too.

Management of ABI challenging behaviour

While a range of factors have a role to play (to a greater or lesser extent) in driving the types of behaviour disorder observed in people with ABI, the reader will be asked to consider that the origin of such problems is almost certainly the product of complex and sometimes bewildering interactions between various contributory variables. Whilst individuals may exhibit similar challenging behaviour, this may be the product of a single causal variable, or any combination of several variables. The nature and interplay of these causes spans many different therapeutic disciplines, requiring clinicians to work together in order to assess and manage the drivers of challenging behaviour effectively.

These subjects are the main substance and concern of this volume. Given diverse causes of behaviour change, a broad range of management options have been utilised, principally drawn from pharmacological and psychological interventions (Rao and Lyketsos, 2000).

The use of approaches drawn from learning theory, especially operant learning, have received much attention in the rehabilitation literature in the past four decades, although its application in neurorehabilitation is much older (Wilson, 1989). There are many advantages to using this approach in both management of challenging behaviour and in regaining or acquiring compensatory skills to counter diminished function arising from ABI (see Alderman, 2001). It is beyond the scope of this volume to provide a detailed comparison of all the available approaches (see Alderman, 2004, for a summary of these), however the best evidence base is obtained by using methods and procedures drawn from learning theory. This especially meets the needs of TBI survivors for whom engagement in 'talking therapies', such as cognitive behaviour therapy, is undermined by lack of awareness, poor motivation, cognitive impairment and challenging behaviour.

One important advantage concerns the challenge of identifying what factors underpin behaviour change. Early proponents supporting the use of methods from learning theory argued that, for the process of assessment, the brain should be considered a dependent variable subjected to environmental manipulation, and the effects studied. In this way, using an inductive approach that stresses objectivity, the nature of the causative factors that underlie behaviour change is more likely to be determined and understood (Wood, 1990).

Consequently, the principal orientation taken in this volume is that of employing learning theory to provide a conceptual framework to assess and understand the complexities of why people behave as they do post-ABI and to provide a means of managing this. Whilst, ultimately, most of the changes observed are an expression of organic damage to neural systems, this is further shaped through post-injury learning and environmental influences, and practices and methods evolved from learning theory and associated frameworks are well placed to identify and counter these. The use of a framework for assessment and management of challenging behaviour is also inclusive, as other methods of change can be incorporated as fits the unique interaction of causal factors for an individual identified from assessment – for example, methods drawn from learning theory combined with medication to counter the neurological causes and post-injury learning that maintain some types of aggressive behaviour disorder (Eames, 1988).

Summary and practical implications

ABI is associated with a wide range of diverse outcomes, including behaviour change, which has various characteristics regarding form, prevalence and impact. This includes absence of purposeful behaviour at one extreme, and tangible risk of serious harm to people at the other. In between these extremes fall a plethora of other behaviours, some of which can be easily described, such as inappropriate sexual behaviour, and others that are idiosyncratic, that are grouped together for convenience – for example, as 'difficulties with social behaviour'. The research literature regarding behaviour outcomes lacks consistency, not least because of lack of standardised definitions of what constitutes behaviour change. However, it is clear that the presence of challenging behaviour has the greatest impact in reducing the autonomy of ABI survivors and potentially has devastating consequences. Neurobehavioural outcomes after severe ABI are often chronic with little prospect of remediation without intervention.

Not all behaviour change is associated with the most disastrous of consequences or warrants clinical intervention. Trying to get a sense of the extent of challenging behaviour that fulfils both these criteria from the literature is difficult, and yet clinicians are routinely confronted with this issue. Sources of bias and the absence of a consensus on terminology affects clinical decision making, which is further complicated by the need to also consider context, cultural norms, pre-morbid personality, and prevailing legislation for the individual case. In terms of practical advice, the authors suggest a good starting point for clinical teams is to agree and adopt a definition of what constitutes challenging behaviour, such as that described above, which can generate a useful set of initial questions as a starting point in discussions regarding whether intervention is appropriate.

This volume is concerned with practical guidance on management of challenging behaviour, a skilled endeavour that is not for the faint-hearted due to the complex nature of neurobehavioural disorder, with behaviour being driven by a variety of factors even when the outward manifestation appears similar, necessitating different approaches to management. The authors advocate that this daunting task is best approached by employing a practical framework drawn from learning theory, which provides a structure within which behavioural symptoms of NBD can be assessed and hypotheses constructed regarding causation, and from these appropriate means of intervention designed, implemented and evaluated, all with the intent of reducing challenging behaviour and increasing personal autonomy and quality of life. This model will now be fully described and explained in the second chapter of this volume.

References

Alderman, N. (2001). Management of challenging behaviour. In R.Ll. Wood and T. McMillan (eds), *Neurobehavioural Disability and Social Handicap Following Traumatic Brain Injury*. Hove: Psychology Press.

Alderman, N. (2003). Rehabilitation of behaviour disorders. In B.A. Wilson (ed.), *Neuropsychological Rehabilitation: Theory and Practice*. Lisse, Netherlands: Swets and Zeitlinger.

Alderman, N. (2004). Disorders of behaviour. In J. Ponsford (ed.), *Cognitive and Behavioural Rehabilitation*. New York: The Guilford Press.

Alderman, N. (2017). Interventions for challenging behaviour. In T. McMillan and R.Ll. Wood (eds), *Neurobehavioural Disability and Social handicap Following Traumatic Brain Injury* (2nd edn). Abingdon: Routledge.

Alderman, N., Williams, C., Knight, C. and Wood, R.Ll. (2017). Measuring change in symptoms of neurobehavioural disability: Responsiveness of the St Andrew's–Swansea Neurobehavioural Outcomes Scale (SASNOS). *Archives of Clinical Neuropsychology*, *32* (8), 951–962.

Alderman, N., Williams, C. and Wood, R.Ll. (2021). Using the St Andrew's–Swansea Neurobehavioural Outcome Scale (SASNOS) to determine prevalence and predictors of neurobehavioural disability among survivors with traumatic brain injury in the community. *Neuropsychological Rehabilitation*. Advance online publication, 28 June 2021. https://doi.org/10.1080/09602011.2021.1946092

Alderman, N., Wood, R.Ll. and Williams, C. (2011). The development of the St Andrew's–Swansea Neurobehavioural Outcome Scale: Validity and reliability of a new measure of neurobehavioural disability and social handicap. *Brain Injury*, *25*, 83–100.

All-Party Parliamentary Group on Acquired Brain Injury (2018). *Time for Change: All-Party Parliamentary Group on Acquired Brain Injury Report*. United Kingdom Acquired Brain Injury Forum: London. https://www.ukabif.org.uk/campaigns/appg-report/

Baguley, I.J., Cooper, J. and Felmingham, K. (2006). Aggressive behaviour following traumatic brain injury: How common is common? *Journal of Head Trauma Rehabilitation*, *21*, 45–56.

Bezeau, S.C., Bogod, N.M. and Mateer, C.A. (2004). Sexually intrusive behaviour following brain injury: Approaches to assessment and rehabilitation. *Brain Injury*, *18*, 299–313.

Broe, A. et al. (1981). The nature and effects of brain damage following severe head injury in young subjects. In T.A.R. Dining and T.J. Connelly (eds.), *Head Injuries* (pp. 92–97), Brisbane: Wiley. Reprinted in part in K.W. Walsh (1985), *Understanding Brain Damage: A Primer of Neuropsychological Evaluation* (p. 145). London: Churchill Livingstone.

Brooks, N., Campsie, L., Symington, C., Beattie, A. and McKinlay, W. (1986). The five year outcome of severe blunt head injury: A relative's view. *Journal of Neurology, Neurosurgery and Psychiatry*, *49*, 764–770.

Dunn, L., Henry, J. and Beard, D. (2003). Social deprivation and adult head injury: A national study. *Journal of Neurology, Neurosurgery and Psychiatry*, *740*, 1060–1064.

Eames, P (1988). Behavior disorders after severe brain injury: Their nature, causes and strategies for management. *Journal of Head Trauma Rehabilitation*, *3*, 1–6.

Emerson, E., Barrett, S., Bell, C., Cummings, R., McCool, C., Toogood, A. and Mansell, J. (1987). *Developing Services for People with Severe Learning Difficulties and Challenging Behaviours*. Canterbury: University of Kent at Canterbury, Institute of Social and Applied Psychology.

Johnson, C., Knight, C. and Alderman, N. (2006). Challenges associated with the definition and assessment of inappropriate sexual behaviour amongst individuals with a neurological impairment. *Brain Injury*, *20*, 687–693.

Johnson, R. and Balleny, H. (1996). Behaviour problems after brain injury: Incidence and need for treatment. *Clinical Rehabilitation*, *10*, 173–181.

Kelly, G., Todd, J., Simpson, G., Kremer, P. and Martin, C. (2006). The Overt Behavior Scale (OBS): A tool for measuring challenging behaviors following ABI in community settings. *Brain Injury*, *20*, 307–319.

Oddy, M., Cattran, C. and Wood, R.Ll. (2008). The development of a measure of motivational changes following acquired brain injury. *Journal of Clinical and Experimental Neuropsychology*, *30*, 568–575.

Oddy, M., Moir, J.F., Fortescue, F. and Chadwick, F. (2010). The prevalence of traumatic brain injury in the homeless community in a UK city. *Brain Injury*, *26*, 1058–1064.

Rabinowitz, A.R. and Levin, H.S. (2014). Cognitive sequelae of traumatic brain injury. *Psychiatric Clinics of North America*, *37*, 1–11.

Rao, V.R. and Lyketsos, M.D. (2000). Neuropsychiatric sequelae of traumatic brain injury. *Psychosomatics*, *41*, 95–103.

Sabaz, M., Simpson, G.K., Alexandra, J.W., Rogers, J.M., Gillis, I. and Strettles, B. (2014). Prevalence, comorbidities, and correlates of challenging behaviour among community-dwelling adults with severe traumatic brain injury: A multicenter study. *Journal of Head Trauma Rehabilitation*, *29*, 19–30.

Starkstein, S.E. and Robinson, R.G. (1991). The role of the human lobes in affective disorder following stroke. In H.S. Levin, H.M. Eisenberg and A.L. Benton (eds), *Frontal Lobe Function and Dysfunction* (pp. 288–303). Oxford: Oxford University Press.

Stéfan, A., Mathé, J. and SOFMER group (2016). What are the disruptive symptoms of behavioural disorders after traumatic brain injury? A systematic review leading to recommendations for good practices. *Annals of Physical and Rehabilitation Medicine*, *59*, 5–17.

Tam, S., McKay, A., Sloan, S. and Ponsford, J. (2015). The experience of challenging behaviours following severe TBI: A family perspective. *Brain Injury*, *29*, 813–821.

Tateno, A., Jage, R.E. and Robinson, R.G. (2003). Clinical correlates of aggressive behavior after traumatic brain injury. *Journal of Neuropsychiatry and Clinical Neurosciences*, *15*, 155–160.

Timmer, M.L., Jacobs, B., Schonherr, M.C., Spikeman, J.M. and Van Der Naalt, J. (2020). The spectrum of long-term behavioural disturbances and provided care after traumatic brain injury. In J.M. Spikeman, J. Van Der Naalt, D. Neumann and M.V. Milders (eds), *Neurobehavioural Changes After Acquired Brain Injury*. Lausanne: Frontiers Media SA. DOI: 10.3389/978-2-88963-955-7

Walsh, K.W. (1985). *Understanding brain damage: A primer for neuropsychological evaluation*. New York: Churchill Livingston.

Williams, W.H. (2012). Repairing shattered lives: Brain injury and its implications for the criminal justice system. Report published by the Barrow Cadbury Trust on behalf of the Transition to Adulthood Alliance. Retrieved from http://yss.org.uk/wp-content/uploads/2012/10/Repairing-Shattered-Lives_Report.pdf

Wilson, B.A. (1989). Behaviour therapy in the treatment of neurologically impaired adults. In P.R. Martin (ed.), *Handbook of Behaviour Therapy and Psychological Science: An Integrative Approach*. New York: Pergamon Press.

Winslade, W. (1999). *Confronting Traumatic Brain Injury: Devastation, Hope and Healing*. London and New Haven, CT: Yale University Press.

Wood, R.Ll. (1990). Conditioning procedures in brain injury rehabilitation. In R.Ll. Wood (ed.), *Neurobehavioural Sequelae of Traumatic Brain Injury* (pp. 153–174). Hove: Psychology Press.

Wood, R.Ll. (2001). Understanding neurobehavioral disability. In R.Ll. Wood and T. McMillan (eds), *Neurobehavioral Disability and Social Handicap Following Traumatic Brain Injury* (pp. 3–27). Hove: Psychology Press.

Worthington, A., Wood, R.Ll. and McMillan, T.M. (2017). Neurobehavioural disability over the past four decades. In T. McMillan and R.Ll. Wood (eds), *Neurobehavioural Disability and Social Handicap Following Traumatic Brain Injury* (2nd edn) (pp. 3–14). Abingdon: Routledge.

2   The intervention model

Frameworks, principles and practice

Nick Alderman

Introduction

As we learned in Chapter 1, the complexities of ABI typically result in multi-variate drivers underpinning challenging behaviour. This mitigates against a universal taxonomy and a prescriptive catalogue of standardised interventions. Instead, drawing from a knowledge base of ABI contributory causal factors and primary methods of intervention from learning theory, behaviour support plans must always be specifically designed to meet the unique needs and circumstances of the individual. A practical alternative to choosing from a pre-scribed range of interventions is the enablement of identifying effective solutions to individual needs through use of a structured framework that facilitates and guides the clinical process. Core features of such a framework are a structured approach to assessment, including identification of variables underpinning challenging behaviour, a means of managing clinical decision making, and the ability to evaluate effectiveness and outcomes. An example of such a framework was originally described by the author (Alderman, 2001) and, since then, this has gone through several revisions and refinements. It comprises what the author refers to as a process model and incorporates several key sequential steps to be followed in order to construct a bespoke behaviour support plan that meets the desired goal. The most recent iteration of this model forms the basis of the current chapter. A major benefit is that it encourages a systematic, objective approach to the management of challenging behaviour, with the further benefit of generating evidence-based outcomes.

The process model draws from three key influences which together underpin its construction and the activities undertaken within each stage. It is necessary for the reader to have some knowledge of these influences to understand the purpose of each stage, including the necessity to follow each step in turn, and to understand the basic principles underpinning the methods from new learning that form the basis of the behaviour support plan it drives (these are illustrated throughout this volume); the array of methods available to the clinician for this purpose are described in Chapter 6.

These key influences will now be described briefly.

DOI: 10.4324/9781003083290-3

Key influence 1: Learning theory

Theories of learning provide conceptual frameworks that describe how new knowledge and skills are acquired. These theories generate specific principles that influence the learning process, and it is from these that practical means of intervention are drawn, resulting in a plan whose goal is behaviour change.

It is beyond the scope of this volume to consider a detailed explanation of the many different types of learning theory, although in neurorehabilitation three have special merit.

Procedural learning

The first is *procedural learning*. This represents the most primitive form of learning and is based on acquiring skills through repeated performance and practice. It has special relevance in neurorehabilitation as neurocognitive impairment that is especially characteristic of TBI (deficits in information processing, attention, memory and the executive functions) mediate conscious learning, such as acquiring new verbal information; when present, these will impede learning via this route to some extent, rendering the learning process slow, variable and sensitive to interference. In contrast, procedural learning, which is often referred to as 'knowing by doing', takes place through frequent, regular repetition of the desired skill, often over a prolonged period, until it becomes ingrained as a habit. This learning theory is especially relevant to people with gross cognitive impairment. Whilst it is most associated with acquiring new motor skills as habits, such as re-learning hygiene skills, it has also been used as a means of successfully reducing challenging behaviour; for example, Alderman and Burgess (1994) reported employing procedural learning methods in the reduction of verbal aggression in the case of a man who presented with a severe global amnesia.

Errorless learning

The second learning theory to consider is that of *errorless learning*. Under this scheme, opportunities to make errors in the learning process are minimised, resulting in faster acquisition of new skills and knowledge, that is less subject to interference and more resilient once the formal learning process has been withdrawn. In neurorehabilitation, it is often used in conjunction with procedural learning. For example, a motor skill to acquire is broken down into a sequence of steps that are practised every day – the procedural learning element. To guide a person through such a sequence, a therapist will deliver a prompt (which can be verbal, physical or both) that the person then follows to ensure successful completion of each task-part in turn – the errorless learning element of the intervention. In this way, the individual avoids errors made by wrongly guessing task-parts, resulting in a successful outcome. It also can be effectively employed in the management of challenging behaviour, especially when this is a function of low frustration-tolerance, when a person is uncertain what to do or makes mistakes, as interventions using, for example, a sequential series of verbal prompts will guide a person through a task while minimising the opportunities in which errors are made, removing potential sources of frustration.

Operant learning

The third theory of learning to consider here is *operant learning*. This has particular relevance in facilitating understanding of post-ABI challenging behaviours, their assessment and management.

Operant learning (also referred to as operant conditioning and instrumental learning), is a theory that predicts behaviour change primarily because of the impact, or consequences, that behaviour has on the environment. Its principles were first explored by Edward Thorndike and then subsequently in greater detail by B.F. Skinner. The basic premise is that all behaviour has an impact in operating on the environment; and that the nature of the consequences resulting from this will influence the likelihood the same behaviour will be repeated. At its simplest level, behaviour always results in one of three consequences for its perpetrator: something pleasant happens; something unpleasant occurs; or there are no obvious consequences, either pleasant or unpleasant.

This deceptively simple theory is underpinned by the discovery and scientifically validated demonstration of how different consequences influence behaviour change; and, emerging from this, the variety of practical methods that have evolved that can be deliberately employed to effect learning.

Again, space available in this volume does not enable a detailed account of operant learning; instead, the interested reader is directed to works concerned exclusively with this subject (e.g., Blackman, 2018) including accounts of some of the earliest reported applications to challenging behaviour following acquired brain injury (e.g., Wood and Eames, 1981; Wood, 1987).

However, an understanding of certain core principles is essential for our purpose, and these will now be explored briefly.

Behaviour results in pleasant consequences

Behaviour that brings about outcomes that are pleasant and enjoyable are rewarded through gratification. The learning outcome of this is that the behaviour is more likely to occur again in future in order to re-experience this reward. Under operant learning theory, behaviour that is rewarded is *reinforced*, and this takes two forms. *Positive reinforcement*: behaviour is more likely to occur again as it results in pleasant consequences for the individual. For example, for a person who enjoys pizza, the behaviour of 'pizza buying' increases when the provider has a two-for-one sale; under these conditions, 'buying behaviour' is positively reinforced. *Negative reinforcement*: behaviour is more likely to be repeated when it results in something unpleasant being removed. For example, when raining, the behaviour of 'using an umbrella' is negatively reinforced as it stops the person from getting wet.

It is important to understand that both types of reinforcement lead to an increase in the particular behaviour, and that both desirable and undesirable behaviours can be rewarded. Two examples of how challenging behaviour can typically be reinforced and encouraged in neurorehabilitation settings will now be considered.

In the first example, consider individuals with reduced frustration-tolerance thresholds. Subsequent weakening of inhibitory control may lead to spontaneous expression of frustration through behaviours that include shouting, screaming or worse because their needs are not being met quickly enough. When carers respond to this behaviour, rehabilitation participants may learn that the deliberate expression of these behaviours provides a means of getting their needs met quickly; when this is the case, these behaviours are repeated and are positively reinforced. The behaviour of carers may also inadvertently contribute. For example, carers dislike shouting and screaming, so they intervene and disrupt these behaviours by giving the participant whatever it is they are demanding. Shouting and screaming are positively reinforced for the participant as the consequence is that their needs are met; however, learning in this context is not limited to rehabilitation participants, carers and clinicians learn behaviour change too. The behaviour set used to interrupt challenging behaviour and meeting the participants needs is also more likely to be repeated in future as it results in an escape from challenging behaviour, that is, it is negatively reinforced. This example makes the point that behaviour has consequences not just for the individual expressing it, but for others in the environment too; and that learning and maintenance of challenging behaviour is a product of complex interactions in the environment. Accordingly, it must be remembered that when planning rehabilitation interventions for challenging behaviour, all operant contingencies maintaining it need to be considered, and the goal for behaviour change inevitably extends beyond the rehabilitation participant.

Next, a second example illustrates how operant learning may result in lack of access to therapy in rehabilitation. Consider physiotherapy. People with ABI may benefit considerably by participating in physiotherapy, but this may be demanding and uncomfortable for some. Individuals may lack insight and fail to fully comprehend the benefits participating in therapy will bring; they may also present with lowered frustration-tolerance thresholds, as in the earlier example. A spontaneous response to discomfort they are unable to supress could be shouting or even aggression. Consequently, the ABI participant learns that shouting and aggression can result in escape from, or avoidance of, an activity for which they fail to comprehend the long-term benefit, as well as the discomfort associated with this activity. Subsequently these challenging behaviours are more likely to be deliberately initiated when invited to physiotherapy. A further consequence might be that therapeutic demands are withdrawn; when the participant repeats this behaviour intentionally to avoid or escape from what they see as an unnecessary, high-demand task, then it is said to have been negatively reinforced. As in the previous example, consequences for behaviour are not limited to the perpetrator, which in the case of challenging behaviour often further creates conditions that inadvertently help maintain it. In this example, the behaviour of giving therapeutic input to an aggressive participant is withdrawn because it results in consequences for the physiotherapist that are aversive. They are less likely to initiate therapeutic activity with the participant in future, because that behaviour resulted in *positive punishment*, a type of learning we will explore briefly below.

Behaviour results in unpleasant consequences

This may take multiple forms, the most relevant for our purpose being *extinction* and *punishment*.

Extinction is the process of learning that takes place when a reinforcer that has been identified as maintaining a behaviour is withdrawn. It is unpleasant for the individual in the sense that the gratification or function the behaviour served is no longer available. The theory predicts that when a reinforcer is consistently made unavailable over time, the behaviour it previously maintained will end as it becomes functionally redundant. When this happens, extinction is said to have occurred and new ways of attempting to fulfil whatever purpose that behaviour had will be sought. This gives the clinical team an opportunity to replace challenging behaviour with an adaptive behaviour or skill that meets that need instead.

It should be noted that, when using extinction to obtain behaviour change, the frequency and/or severity of that behaviour is likely to increase in the first instance, a phenomenon known as an *extinction burst* (Lerman, Iwata and Wallace, 1999). Two points arise from this. The first is that use of extinction in interventions targeting self-harm, such as head banging, or physical aggression against other people, must for obvious reasons be very carefully monitored and carried out with extreme caution. Preferably, an alternative means of intervention should be employed, such as reinforcing increasingly fewer episodes of challenging behaviour over time, or replacing this behaviour with something incompatible with it. The second point is an interesting one in that inexperienced clinicians and carers who report an increase in challenging behaviour during the early part of an intervention employing extinction will also often conclude the plan is not working and advocate an alternative approach be employed. Paradoxically, this observation is likely to be a positive indication that the intervention is having the desired effect, and if the temporary increase in behaviour can be tolerated and is safe, the plan should be maintained.

A point regarding good practice when employing extinction is that, whenever possible, efforts are also made to positively reinforce other, desirable behaviours. An example of this in practice is described in Chapter 6, which considers how behaviour support interventions are employed in the management of aggressive behaviour that prevents engagement in neurorehabilitation.

Punishment is the second operant learning principle concerned with unpleasant consequences following behaviour. Behaviours that are punished are less likely to be exhibited again. Punishment takes two forms, *positive punishment* and *negative punishment*. Both positive and negative punishment will always decrease behaviour. The difference between the two is that positive punishment yields an unpleasant, aversive consequence for behaviour, while negative punishment results in something the individual finds pleasurable being removed.

The principle of punishment can help explain the reasons why post-ABI individuals engage in challenging behaviour and underpin interventions to manage it. Positive punishment can often account for the reasons individuals are excluded from therapy. For example, efforts to deliver therapeutic activity by clinicians may result in learning by positive punishment as the outcome is that challenging behaviour is directed at them, including being shouted at, verbally abused and physically assaulted. When these unpleasant consequences exceed the threshold of acceptance held by an individual clinician, they learn not to engage individuals in therapeutic activity in order to avoid these consequences. Examples of the use of positive punishment in attempts to bring about behaviour change are endemic in the early behaviour modification literature, including from neurorehabilitation (see Wood, 1987). However, in contemporary times interventions utilising positive punishment should never be employed, both for ethical reasons and because of the finding that, whilst aversive consequences to behaviour may quickly lead to its reduction, any benefits arising from this are quickly reversed.

Whilst positive punishment can provide a means of explaining how the behaviour of clinicians and care givers inadvertently creates conditions in which challenging behaviour is maintained, negative punishment is more likely to be used as a means of ethically and effectively managing such behaviour. Interventions that result in something of value being lost contingent on challenging behaviour taking place are not uncommon, often when reinforcement strategies have not proved effective or not been indicated, and the reader is referred to Chapter 6 regarding this.

Behaviour has no consequence

Upon first thought, this contingency seems unlikely, certainly within the context of a busy neurorehabilitation environment where challenging behaviour is likely to elicit responses from people, be they staff, other rehabilitation participants, family members or visitors. Causing no response whatever, in conjunction with routine reinforcement of all desirable behaviour, would be the ideal way of preventing the development of challenging behaviour, but outside the confines of a highly specialised neurobehavioural rehabilitation facility, this is improbable.

However, it is worth noting that, in certain circumstances, there may be no obvious impact to the external environment of some challenging behaviour and an absence of external reinforcers or punishers. These include times when the rehabilitation participant is alone, or in cases where they may be isolated from the external world through, for example, disorders of consciousness. When this is the case, the ongoing presence of challenging behaviour may be serving some self-stimulating function, such as might be the case with self-injurious behaviours, and the challenging behaviour is maintained by a process of automatic reinforcement.

Multiple determinants of behaviour

To recap, operant learning theory maintains all behaviour has consequences, and the nature of these consequence is a powerful determinant of whether behaviours are repeated. They are more likely to be repeated if they result in something pleasant, desirable (reinforcement: positive and negative). Conversely, they are less likely to be repeated if they comprise new behaviours that do not result in reinforcement, or, if already part of a behavioural repertoire, the expected reward is withdrawn (extinction), or if the consequence elicited is aversive, unpleasant (punishment: positive and negative).

Of course, behaviour change is potentially a function of multiple drivers that further influence the learning process and that will also need to be considered. Due to the complexities of ABI, the presence of multiple drivers of challenging behaviour frequently results in behaviour support plans that combine as many of the intervention methods described in Chapter 6 as necessary. The point was made earlier that only considering the contingencies operating on the challenging behaviour of the perpetrator is insufficient, and that those operating on other people also require exploration to achieve proper understanding of how and why behaviour is maintained. Table 2.1 summarises the operators contributing to two major categories of challenging behaviour observed in neurorehabilitation settings: 'need gratification', where poorly controlled and impulsive behaviours that result in need gratification for the ABI participant are maintained by both positive and negative reinforcement; and a collection of 'anti-rehabilitation' behaviours leading to cessation of therapeutic input that are sustained through both negative reinforcement and positive punishment. Working out the relationships between behavioural contingencies provides both a means of understanding why rehabilitation participants behave as they do and how carers can inadvertently also contribute to this process.

In addition to environmental influences and post-injury learning, challenging behaviour conceptualised as being symptomatic of a broader pattern of changes resulting in neurobehavioural disability may also be the product of interaction with the functional consequences arising from neurological damage (for example, various types of epilepsy, reduced frustration-tolerance threshold), neurocognitive impairment (for example, frustration driven by the consequences of executive function impairment, poor self-monitoring) and exacerbation of negative pre-morbid personality traits (for example, aggression). These additional variables are subject to separate assessment but

Table 2.1 Summary of how operant contingencies operating on both participants and carers (anybody who engages with the former) contributes to the creation and maintenance of challenging behaviour

'NEED GRATIFICATION' – *attention motivated*

Antecedent	*CONSEQUENCE/ FUNCTION Rehab participant behaviour*	*Operant learning*	*CONSEQUENCE/ FUNCTION Carers' behaviour*	*Operant learning*
Participant expresses challenging behaviour	Results in needs being met by carers	Positive reinforce-ment	Carers intervene to meet participants needs – results in cessation of challenging behaviour	Negative reinforce-ment

'ANTI-REHABILITATION' – *escape/avoidance motivated*

Antecedent	*CONSEQUENCE/ FUNCTION Rehab participant behaviour*	*Operant learning*	*CONSEQUENCE/ FUNCTION Carers' behaviour*	*Operant learning*
Carers attempt to engage participant in therapeutic activity	Expresses challenging behaviour – results in avoidance of/ escape from perceived high-demand/ unnecessary activities	Negative reinforce-ment	Carer stops efforts to engage partici-pant in therapeu-tic activity	Positive punishment

factored in with all known operant contingencies to arrive at a formulation regarding causes of behaviour. This will be explored later in the chapter.

A final point to note regarding multiple drivers of behaviour is that of schedules of reinforcement and punishment, that is, when and how often a reinforcer or punisher is delivered and its subsequent impact on learning. These are based on the number of responses (ratio schedule) or time elapsed (interval schedule). In either case, contingencies can be delivered continuously or at fixed or variable intervals. Learning is most likely to take place when contingencies are delivered every time the behaviour of interest occurs; this is the ideal to aim for when implementing an intervention using operant learning techniques. However, in the complexities of the 'real world' with its many potential sources of error, naturally occurring schedules of reinforcement are more likely to be variable or random. A finding of interest arising from the scientific study of operant learning is that this intermittent form of responding to behaviours increases resistance to extinction, a fact that is very important to bear in mind when attempting to change behaviour. It may only take one or two people in a clinical team who reinforce a behaviour to maintain it and undermine an operant learning intervention; maintaining as consistent approach as possible from everybody is highly desirable to prevent this happening. A further point is that the continuous availability of reinforcers can lead to another operant principle taking place, that of *satiation*, the process where repeated, continuous availability of a reinforcer renders it neutral or even aversive. This points to the need for behaviour support plans to move from a continuous schedule of reinforcement – to establish the desired behaviour – to an intermittent or variable schedule – to maintain behaviour change. Satiation can also be employed as a means of establishing desired behaviour change. For example, Alderman (1991) described how it was used in the reduction of challenging behaviour exhibited by a 24-year-old male who had sustained a severe traumatic brain injury that had proved impervious to effective management using medical and other psychological treatments.

Key influence 2: Applied behaviour analysis

The above principles of operant learning, and other learning theories, are employed within the scientific discipline of applied behaviour analysis (ABA) with the goal of achieving behaviour change. ABA replaced the earlier school of Behaviour Modification, as, unlike the former, it explicitly attempts to determine the functional relationship between behaviour and the environment. Determining the contribution of both antecedents and consequences to behaviour can greatly assist in formulating what function it underpins for the individual, and, from this, derive an effective treatment intervention.

Functional assessment (FA), also referred to as functional behaviour assessment (FBA), describes several defined methodologies that have evolved within ABA for this purpose. FA/FBA involves the collection of data, observations and information to develop a clear understanding of the relationship of events and circumstances that trigger and maintain challenging behaviour. There are three principal forms of FA/FBA, all of which can be usefully employed in the context of neurorehabilitation. They will now be briefly described.

Indirect FA/FBA

Under this scheme, information is gathered about challenging behaviour from informants who know the ABI survivor well and, when possible, from the person themselves. Several tools may be used, including perusal of clinical notes and reports, interviewing people, and use of standardised questionnaires and rating scales.

Standardisation of interview protocols using questionnaires, such as the functional assessment interview (O'Neill et al., 1997) are quick to administer and provide a wide range of information. However, relying on testimony from others should not be the sole source from which information is generated about behaviour, as individual recall is susceptible to bias and error. Use of rating scales can reduce these and provide useful proxy measures of behaviour. Two are especially worthy of note. First, the Overt Behaviour Scale (OBS) (Kelly et al., 2006) was developed to record challenging behaviours displayed by people with TBI. Nine categories of challenging behaviour (various forms of aggression, inappropriate sexual behaviour, perseveration/repetition, wandering/absconding, lack of initiation) are assessed using 34 behavioural descriptors, each of which is rated regarding frequency, severity and the impact it has. Second, the St Andrew's–Swansea Neurobehavioural Outcomes Scale (SASNOS) (Alderman, Wood and Williams, 2011) collates information regarding five principal domains of symptoms of NBD (interpersonal relationships, cognition, inhibition, aggression and communication) through rating the presence and severity of 49 symptoms underpinning these. An important point to emphasise is that both the OBS and SASNOS were specifically conceptualised and designed for use in TBI, as opposed to being instruments imported from general psychiatry that are assumed to work as intended with this clinical group. They are straightforward to administer and score, provide a profile of strengths and weaknesses, and have known psychometric properties, enabling them to make valuable contributions to assessment, formulation and outcome measurement.

Observational FA/FBA

Indirect functional assessment methods involve gathering data from which function can be inferred. In contrast, direct functional assessment approaches use formalised observation to generate correlational evidence of causal relationships between possible environmental variables with behaviour.

A popular direct functional assessment approach is *observational FA/FBA*, which collects data used to construct a descriptive assessment of behaviour. Behaviour is directly observed, as discreetly as possible; when behaviours of interest take place, the observer records information about this and the circumstances in which it took place, including antecedents and consequences. The extent of the information collected is defined in advance, varying from freehand accounts of variables of note, through to use of observational recording measures (ORM), comprising highly sophisticated information-gathering instruments with known psychometric properties that minimise observer bias and error and produce a number of quantifiable indices. Periods of observation also vary. This can be continuous – any time an ABI participant engages in a defined behaviour, a record of this is made by whichever staff member observed it. Alternatively, data collection may be restricted to defined periods through a procedure called time-sampling. The range of options for collecting observational data, and reasons underpinning these, are discussed in Chapter 5.

Data generated using observational FA/FBA can provide a highly objective means of determining relationships between behaviour and the environment. The information is also quantitative in that frequency counts of behaviour, and the different antecedents and consequences, are collected, enabling statistical and other means of analysis to be utilised. For example, *conditional probability* *analysis* can be performed, indicating which events are most likely to be associated with the challenging behaviour. As an example, indices that describe possible relationships between a range of observed antecedents to behaviour can be constructed using the formula (frequency antecedent co-occurring with behaviour/total frequency of behaviour) *100. Resultant indices corresponding to the complete range of antecedents observed can then be compared to arrive at a quantitative appreciation of those most likely to have a meaningful relationship in the maintenance of that behaviour, as opposed to preceding it by chance or being recorded in error.

Functional analysis/experimental functional analysis

The second most well-known form of direct approach is *functional analysis* (FAn), also referred to as *experimental functional analysis* (EFAn).

FAn/EFAn involves the systematic manipulation of environmental conditions in an artificial setting, to identify the variables that control and maintain challenging behaviours. Experimental control is deemed to be evident when a change in condition brings an associated change in behaviour. In scientific parlance, challenging behaviour is deemed the equivalent of the dependent variable, whilst different environmental variables are assigned the role of independent variables that are systematically and separately introduced to determine what influence they have on the dependent variable, and this is measured. Assessment is conducted in a physical space in which the assessors have as much control as possible to minimise error attributable to other factors, in order to determine the influence of variables of interest reliably. This highly objective approach to assessment has the advantage of scientific determinism in proving relationships between environmental conditions and behaviour, unlike the indirect and observational forms assessment described above, which comprise descriptive analysis methodologies only capable of generating correlational evidence of associations.

Several decades of research has established that FAn/EFAn is an effective means of determining the function of challenging behaviour and its management (Beavers, Iwata and Lerman, 2013). Although in theory there are no restrictions on what environmental factors are introduced as independent variables, a typical assessment utilises contingencies serving reward, avoidance/escape and automatic reinforcement functions and compares the frequency/severity of challenging behaviour elicited by each of these with a control condition. These are operationalised as follows:

Attention

Is challenging behaviour rewarded by attention? Attention, often in the form of comments condemning challenging behaviour, is only given as a consequence of this behaviour.

Demand

Is challenging behaviour a means of avoiding or escaping from a demanding activity? A high-demand task is introduced and removed immediately contingent on challenging behaviour.

Tangible

Is challenging behaviour a function of obtaining desired items? Preferred items are made available to the person immediately after they engage in challenging behaviour.

Alone

Does challenging behaviour serve a self-stimulation function? The person is placed in a low-stimulation environment, when challenging behaviour occurs in the absence of any obvious antecedent or consequence, suggesting that the reward is internal and cannot be directly observed. When this is the case, assumed self-stimulation results in what is referred to as automatic reinforcement.

Control

A comparison or baseline condition in which challenging behaviour is least likely to occur. A favoured activity is undertaken, punctuated with regular, positive interaction with staff.

None of the above forms of assessment are mutually exclusive. For example, observational FA/FBA can be continuously maintained within a clinical environment, with recordings being made whenever challenging behaviour takes place. Indirect methods may be used concurrently, where information from the historical and clinical records, interviews and questionnaire and rating scales, generates further information to enrich and supplement direct observational measures. These assessments may generate a range of hypotheses concerning relationships between environmental factors and challenging behaviour, which can be rigorously examined by conducting a functional/experimental functional analysis.

Structured descriptive assessment

A final point to consider in this section is that of a more recent development, the *structured descriptive assessment*, which combines the advantages offered by both descriptive and experimental methodologies, into a single hybrid assessment (Freeman, Anderson and Scotti, 2000). Several disadvantages and conceptual, ethical and practical limitations have been raised regarding the previous methods; for example, the weaker, correlational evidence of environmental-behavioural relationships from descriptive methods, and the potential detrimental impact from changing context and delivering contingencies to behaviour using unfamiliar staff in experimental analysis (Lerman and Iwata, 1993). In contrast, structured descriptive assessment has been reported as having potentially the most to offer management of ABI challenging behaviour. First, it involves the systematic presentation of different classes of antecedent events that relate to behavioural function. This feature partly resembles the rationale of an experimental functional analysis. However, unlike the experimental model, consequences are not manipulated in a structured descriptive assessment but instead naturally occurring responses transpire. Second, it is conducted in the natural environment by typical care providers. This feature resembles a descriptive assessment and contrasts with an experimental functional analysis, which involves artificial settings and unknown experimenters. Although not widely reported, evidence suggests the utility of structured descriptive assessment in management of brain injury mediated challenging behaviour, including time required to conduct an assessment. For example, Rahman, Alderman and Oliver (2013) used this approach in investigations of challenging behaviour in four people with acquired brain injury. A principal advantage was in terms of efficiency: a reliable measure of functional relationships was obtained with a mean assessment duration of just 2.25 hours per person.

Key influence 3: Single case study experimental design methodology

The final framework that makes an important contribution to the practical model subsequently to be described (that will provide a means of guiding and facilitating behaviour support plans) is single case experimental design (SCED) methodology.

SCED provides a wealth of approaches that were applied from the middle of the last century, following criticism that clinical procedures used at the time were largely unproven. Accordingly, clinicians began to incorporate scientific methods into their clinical work and, therefore, contribute to practice-based research to improve the quality and effectiveness of psychological interventions. Adopting a research-based approach to practice enabled, for the first time, the objective evaluation of clinical applications; the resulting quantification of psychological concepts and measurement of behaviour change were key features of early behaviourism and the subsequent transformation of psychology as a science.

The core feature of SCED has already been described in relation to FAn/EFAn earlier: the ability to articulate and isolate behaviour of interest and to determine the effect of various treatment interventions on it, in conditions that minimise sources of error that might otherwise undermine this process. In its simplest form, the behaviour of interest is measured for a period of time under the same conditions; this comprises a baseline, that is, a quantifiable description of what comprises the behaviour, its frequency, and perhaps severity and impact. Challenging behaviour is rendered the dependent variable, and conditions remain as constant as possible during the baseline stage. It is important that

sufficient measurements are taken to demonstrate that behaviour is not changing and is relatively stable over time. When enough measurements are taken, a
behaviour support plan that articulates what is required is implemented; and
continued measurement of the dependent variable will determine the impact
this has. Over time, a comparison of the baseline and treatment phases will give
an indication of the effectiveness of the independent variable in reducing the
frequency/severity/impact of this behaviour. In the short term, reverting to a
second 'baseline only' phase may result in a subsequent increase in it again,
whilst reintroducing the intervention in a second treatment phase should reverse
this, if the latter is truly an agent of change. Continued measurement of behaviour as the dependent variable under conditions that minimise error, and measurement of 'cause-and-effect' changes to behaviour when interventions are
introduced in a highly controlled way as independent variables, enables very
exact determination and evaluation of their effect. Furthermore, switching an
intervention on and off and observing the effect on behaviour provides a means
of articulating true effectiveness, above the correlational level where this might
still reasonably be attributed to chance, if this were only introduced once.

Convention is for 'no treatment' or baseline conditions to be labelled 'A' and
introduction of successive treatment interventions as 'B', 'C' and so on. Probably the most often utilised SCED methodology is the reversal design, as described
above, where baseline and treatment conditions are successively withdrawn/
introduced to evaluate the latter, comprising the ABAB illustrated in Figure 2.1.

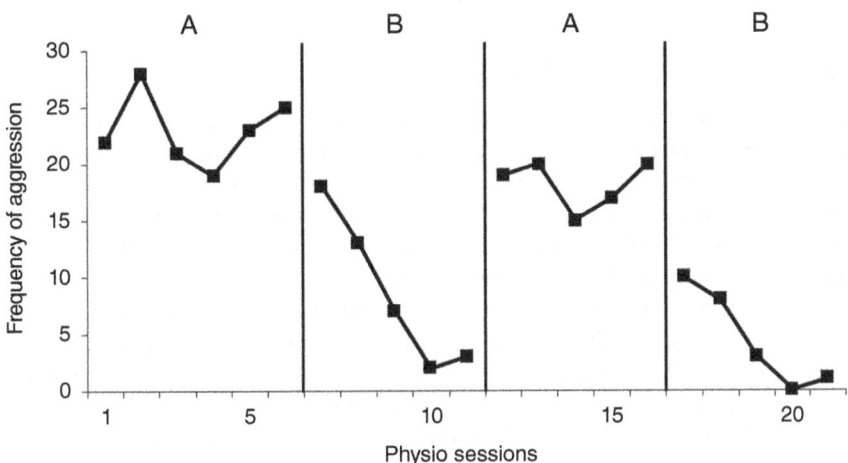

Figure 2.1 An example of an ABAB multiple baseline design to help determine outcome on aggressive behaviour of an individual treatment intervention. Each
data point represents the frequency of defined aggression in a single physiotherapy session. 'A' represents sessions in which there was no treatment intervention in operation (baseline), 'B' represents sessions in which the
intervention was implemented (treatment). Data is fictitious and is for illustrative purposes only.

In conclusion, SCED methodologies provide a practical means of determining the effectiveness of interventions and occupies an important function in our model. SCED methodologies are also especially important in the study and rehabilitation of acquired neurological conditions where lack of homogeneity within clinical populations exerts limitations on the integrity of data when this is pooled (Alderman, 2002). The approaches are very flexible and can be easily designed to meet individual needs while still enabling scientific determination of clinical applications in neurorehabilitation. Examples of the various approaches will be described throughout this volume.

Space in this volume does not enable a detailed description and critique of SCED methodologies; instead, the interested reader is referred to an oft-quoted source now in its third edition (Barlow, Nock and Hersen, 2008), to the specific application to neurorehabilitation settings by the current author (Alderman, 2002) and to a further volume in the current modular handbook series by Tate and Perdices (2019).

A process model to manage decision making in providing behaviour support in ABI

Having considered the three main influences contributing to the model and activities undertaken within it, the framework governing and facilitating clinical activities capable of managing challenging behaviour will now be described. This account needs to be read with reference to the visual descriptions of the model in Figures 2.2 and 2.3.

Step 1: Consideration of ethical and legal issues

Faced with the task of attempting to change an individual's behaviour, the starting point must be *deciding if it is 'right' to intervene* at all. Unfortunately, ABI participants may be unable to provide informed consent if they lack awareness or have poor insight, a finding not unusual in TBI survivors (Cooper-Evans et al., 2008). In addition to constraints imposed by the legislative framework in which clinicians work, (see Chapter 3), a multitude of moral and ethical concerns may be raised about risk and about what constitutes acceptable behaviour, especially within a team-based model of clinical decision making in which personal and professional issues may come to the fore (McGrath, 2007). Tolerance of behaviour varies, depending on a range of factors including age, culture, context in which behaviour occurs, prevailing legislation, local norms and expectations, and the belief structures and values of communities, family members, carers and professionals. Behaviours that increase vulnerability, limit or delay access to community resources, and decrease likelihood of attaining full rehabilitation potential are likely to require intervention (Alderman 2001). Certain behaviours attract greater consensus that implementing a behaviour support plan is appropriate, including physical aggression and sexual assaults. However, Alderman (2017) found that agreement among

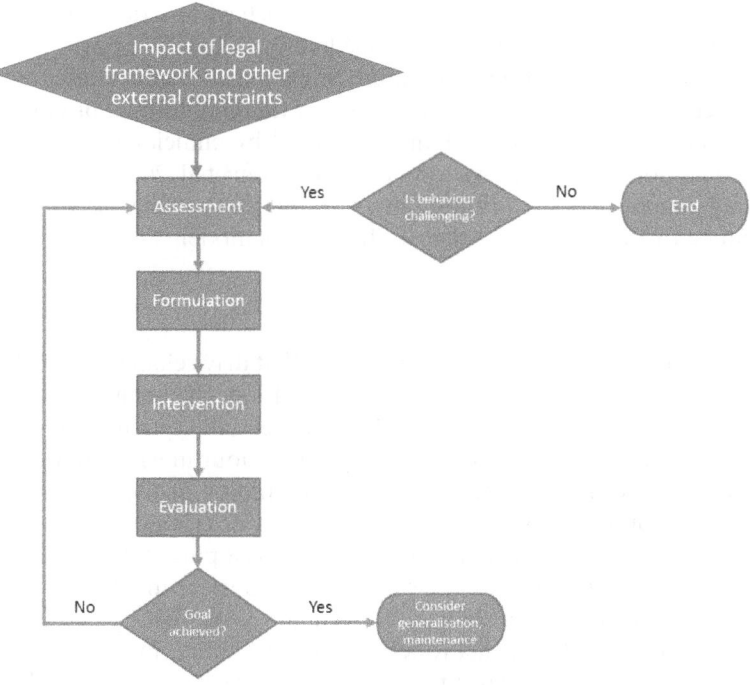

Figure 2.2 Flowchart illustrating a process model to manage implementation of interventions to manage challenging behaviour in acquired brain injury.

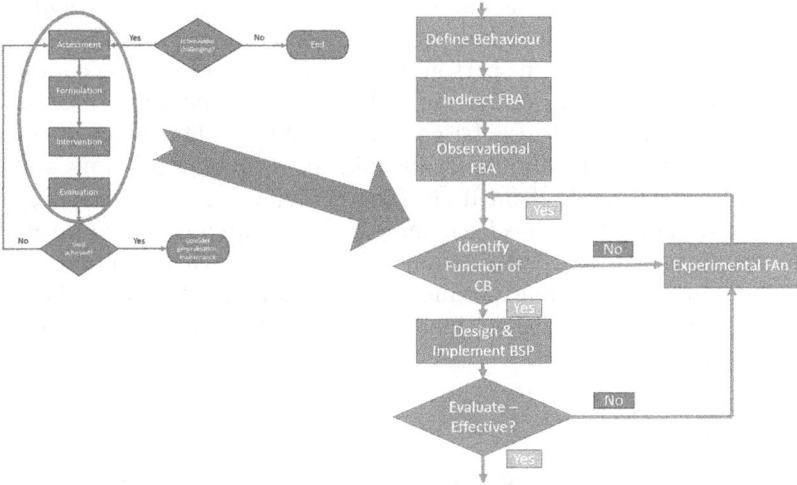

Figure 2.3 Enlargement of the assessment stage in the process model to illustrate usage
of indirect and observational functional assessment and functional analysis
methods.

rehabilitation professionals about a range of behaviours described as 'challenging' in clinical practice varied considerably, which supports the points made earlier about variance in individual thresholds for what constitutes challenging behaviour. Research also suggests that families adopt a broader definition of challenging behaviour than is accepted by clinicians, which includes social, educational and employment outcomes (Tam et al. 2015). Consequently, obtaining consent among all those involved and making the decision to intervene can be the most difficult stage in the process model.

Step 2: Assessment

The next step is *assessment* to identify factors that drive challenging behaviour, to create a formulation regarding its function. First, the behaviour concerned is articulated using objectively defined and observable qualities (see Chapter 5). Second, a detailed functional analysis of behaviour in which information is collected from multiple sources aids an understanding of the need it fulfils for the rehabilitation participant. This will include identifying operant contingencies concerning carers that contribute to its development and maintenance. The principal steps to consider are shown in detail in Figure 2.3. As described earlier, functional analysis provides a proven means of identifying the multiple drivers known to underpin neurobehavioural disability, in conjunction with the outputs from other relevant assessments, especially neuropsychological assessment.

As Figure 2.3 suggests, indirect assessment to identify causal factors driving challenging behaviour should routinely be undertaken from perusal of documents, including historical reports and contemporary clinical records, specialised investigations, including neuropsychological assessments and imaging studies, interviews with family, carers and others who know the rehabilitation participant well, the person themselves, and through the completion of relevant questionnaires and rating scales. Whenever possible, direct observational FA/FBA should also be conducted. Where clinical resources and organisation permits, this should ideally take the form of continuous observation, such that whenever defined challenging behaviours occur, appropriate records (in whatever form has been agreed) (see Chapter 5) are completed. If doubt remains regarding the relationship between environmental variables and behaviour, a functional/experimental analysis should be undertaken, with additional consideration being made towards utilisation of a structured descriptive assessment.

Stage 3: Formulation

Formulation is the creation of hypotheses regarding causes, precipitants and the maintenance of the influences of a person's psychological, interpersonal and behavioural problems (Eells, Kekjelic and Lucas, 1998). This framework is further used to drive the components of the behaviour support plan.

In the context of ABI and the underpinning frameworks outlined earlier, information from multiple sources is integrated to generate a hypothesis about what is driving challenging behaviour, which informs the formulation. For example, aggressive behaviour is frequently found to fulfil an escape or avoidance function in response to therapy demands and is consequently maintained through reinforcement (Alderman, 2007). Table 2.1 gives examples of how knowledge of the different operant contingencies impacting on the perpetrator of challenging behaviour and others in the environment can combine to create and maintain behaviours incompatible with achieving good outcomes in neurorehabilitation.

The formulation will also draw from the findings of the other assessments referred to earlier that provide information about other contributing factors that interact to a variable extent with these contingencies. As an expression of neurobehavioural disability, challenging behaviour may primarily be attributable to one of these drivers, a combination of several, or even all of them. Formulation will necessarily need to consider a comprehensive set of variables to optimise the validity of hypotheses about challenging behaviour. Arriving at a clear understanding of the function of behaviour and how it is maintained will determine the intervention approaches most likely to be effective. Examples of the multifactorial approach to assessment and formulation of challenging behaviour within an operant learning framework will be illustrated throughout this volume.

Stage 4: Intervention

Having arrived at an empirical understanding of the frequency, longevity and prevalence of challenging behaviour, and having created a hypothesis – formulation – of the reasons driving this, the next stage in the model is the design and implementation of a behaviour support plan based on this. Describing specific intervention types in detail is beyond the scope of this chapter: see Chapter 6 for a full account of these methods, together with examples of their use in subsequent chapters. Drawing from the formulation, both environmental manipulation (including modification of antecedents to behaviour) and changing existing contingencies to behaviour, will normally form the basis of the management plan. Examples of contingency management interventions include (but are not limited to) those underpinned by principles of positive and negative reinforcement, extinction and negative punishment (for example, differential reinforcement, shaping, chaining, fading, exposure, time-out, verbal mediation, simplified forms of cognitive-behavioural therapy, and response-cost).

Because of the complex drivers of behaviour and consequent likelihood that multiple reasons account for these, it is usually the case that behaviour support plans incorporate multiple methods, and that these multi-component interventions are the norm. Clinicians should use whatever combination of methods is best suited to meet the needs of the participant as indicated by the formulation. The emphasis should be on promoting independence and autonomy and on optimising consistency by encouraging and rewarding desirable behaviour (positive reinforcement) and 'playing down' behaviour that is not (extinction). In this sense, interventions based on learning theory usually change the behaviour of those charged with the care and rehabilitation of the participant, promoting growth of positive relationships and an enriched social climate, or milieu, that is a necessary condition for the achievement of good rehabilitation outcomes.

A further benefit of using multi-component behaviour support plans drawn from learning theory concerns co-existing forms of neurocognitive impairment, especially memory and executive dysfunction, which in some cases play an important role in driving challenging behaviour and provide challenges to intervention. These can create a range of difficulties, including deficient self-monitoring, in which reduction in the ability to use and respond to feedback from the environment leads to cues being missed and results in so-called 'behavioural perseveration.' These types of impairments explain difficulties in social interaction that often characterise TBI, often described by patients' family members as lack of tact, selfishness or ignorance. In these cases, different patterns of neurocognitive impairment will determine what methods drawn from the three types of learning theory briefly considered at the start of this chapter can be employed effectively to both change behaviour and circumvent difficulties in the learning process itself. These will be considered in detail in subsequent chapters throughout this volume.

Step 5: Evaluation

The final stage is evaluating the effectiveness of the behaviour support plan and, if successful, considering those issues concerning the extent to which this is withdrawn (least restrictive practice).

The application of principles from learning theory into behaviour support plans is a quantitatively driven process, where both assessment and treatment are concerned with objective measurement and determination of cause-and-effect relationships. In the assessment stage, behaviour is first subject to objective definition and examination; it can be unambiguously observed with a high degree of agreement between those persons present, and counted, measured and analysed in efforts to determine prevalence and underlying causes. Conceptualising challenging behaviour as the equivalent of the dependent variable in scientific study does not stop at the assessment stage. As we learned earlier when we considered single case study experimental design methodologies, an advantage of adopting a scientific approach is that reliable, valid data continues to be collected throughout the process. Continuation of this beyond assessment minimises error measurement and enables comparison, enabling precise determination of an intervention on challenging behaviour by comparison of 'no treatment' vs 'treatment', or baseline vs intervention, conditions.

Many of the measurement methods and instruments used in the assessment stage can simply carry on being used for this purpose throughout the life of the behaviour support plan, including those described in detail in Chapter 5 and throughout this volume.

An advantage of continuous data collection is that it can be closely monitored to help clinicians understand if their plan is having the predicted effect or not. In the early days of an intervention, this availability of online monitoring provides information from which the plan can be subjected to precise adjustment and calibration. If data does not fall as predicted, decisions can be taken regarding returning to the assessment and formulation stages to rethink drivers of behaviour and potential challenges to the learning process. If all goes well, monitoring of data regarding the behaviour as the independent variable will support future decision making regarding matters such as generalisation of the gains made for other environments and contexts, moving from a continuous to a variable schedule of reinforcement to avoid satiation, and stopping the intervention completely. In some cases, reducing the components making up a behaviour support plan to the minimum level required may be indicated in order to secure long-term benefits (for example, to circumvent neurocognitive impairment that both drives challenging behaviour and impairs new learning).

Summary and practical implications

Operant learning theory provides a conceptual framework to help understand the evolution and maintenance of challenging behaviour, and a practical role when its underlying principles of mediating behaviour change are used in interventions concerned with their elimination and substitution with adaptive behaviours. Methods evolved in ABA provide a toolkit to determine the functional relationship between behaviour and the environment. Determining the contribution of antecedents to and consequences for behaviour is of great value in identifying the function challenging behaviour underpins, and from this the subsequent design of effective interventions. SCED provides a further framework and toolkit that enables practitioners to effectively design and implement behaviour support plans and gauge their effectiveness. Its methods elevate clinical work to a level compatible with research, enabling an exact understanding of the relative impact of each part of a typical multi-component behaviour support plan and potential contributions to the evidence base regarding its constituent components.

Together, these three influences underpin a practical model that can successfully guide clinicians through the process of facilitating effective strategies in the management of challenging behaviour.

Some practical points arising from this include:

1 Each step of the process intervention model should be worked through methodically and in sequence.
2 It is especially important that sufficient time and energy is spent on working with those concerned, first, in achieving agreement that behaviour is challenging and that clinically/ethically/legally acceptable efforts should be directed at changing it, and, second, that the behaviour is defined using objective, operational criteria so that everybody is in no doubt when it takes place.

3 A shared ethos and responsibility for facilitating behaviour change needs to be developed. Without this joint ownership of the process, inconsistency in agreement that behaviour is challenging, variability in recognition when it takes place, and discrepancy in response to this will undermine new learning and the potential success of the behaviour support plan. A consistent approach by all concerned is paramount.

4 It is vital to remember that challenging behaviour has consequences for all when it takes place, not just the perpetrator. Reinforcement and punishment will impact simultaneously on the rehabilitation participant and others in the environment, carers and other service users. Understanding the impact of all these contingencies, not just those directly affecting the perpetrator, need to be recognised and their contribution to maintaining challenging behaviour assessed. Interventions concerned with behaviour change are not limited to the person who engages in challenging behaviour; changing responses of others concerned with the care of that person is also highly likely.

5 The empirical approach described here makes the point that after a formulation and behaviour support plan have been agreed, assessment and intervention are inseparable. Continuous, ongoing collection of data regarding the dependent variable facilitates ongoing review so that if evidence of behaviour change is not convincing, a return to a further assessment phase can take place and a revised plan subsequently implemented. This cycling between assessment and intervention replicates the SCED multiple design methodology, with a 'no treatment', 'A' stage, being followed by a 'treatment', 'B' stage, and if necessary further variations in the latter designated 'C', 'D' and so on. The detail in Figure 2.3 is especially important. A combination of indirect and observational FA/FBA is often sufficient to generate a robust formulation and treatment plan. However, if a formulation is still lacking, or an intervention unsuccessful, then undertaking a functional analysis/experimental functional analysis as described earlier and illustrated in Figure 2.3 should be considered.

6 Finally, when an intervention is successful, thought must be given to how this is removed. Ideally, the behaviour support plan can be withdrawn and behaviour change maintained without further modification of contingencies and the environment. However, neurocognitive impairment may necessitate it being maintained, or reduced to the minimum to compensate for these difficulties. Thought also has to be given to the behaviour of future carers who will need educating about how to respond to the rehabilitation participant to avoid the subsequent reinforcement of challenging behaviour.

References

Alderman, N. (1991). The treatment of avoidance behaviour following severe brain injury by satiation through negative practice. *Brain Injury*, *5*, 77–86.

Alderman, N. (2001). Management of challenging behaviour. In R.Ll. Wood and T. McMillan (eds), *Neurobehavioural Disability and Social Handicap Following Traumatic Brain Injury*. Hove: Psychology Press.

Alderman, N. (2002). Individual case studies. In S. Priebe and M. Slade (eds). *Evidence in Mental Health Care*. Hove: Brunner-Routledge.

Alderman, N. (2007). Prevalence, characteristics and causes of aggressive behaviour observed within a neurobehavioural rehabilitation service: Predictors and implications for management. *Brain Injury, 21*, 891–911.

Alderman, N. (2017). Interventions for challenging behaviour. In T. McMillan and R.Ll. Wood (eds). *Neurobehavioural Disability and Social Handicap Following Traumatic Brain Injury* (2nd edn). Abingdon: Psychology Press.

Alderman, N. and Burgess, P. (1994). A comparison of treatment methods for behaviour disorders following herpes simplex encephalitis. *Neuropsychological Rehabilitation, 4*, 31–48.

Alderman, N., Wood, R.Ll. and Williams, C. (2011). The development of the St Andrew's–Swansea Neurobehavioural Outcome Scale: Validity and reliability of a new measure of neurobehavioural disability and social handicap. *Brain Injury, 25*, 83–100.

Barlow, D.H., Nock, M.K. and Hersen, M. (2008). *Single Case Experimental Designs: Strategies for Studying Behavior Change* (3rd edn). New York: Allyn & Bacon.

Beavers, G.A., Iwata, B.A. and Lerman, D.C. (2013). Thirty years of research on the functional analysis of problem behavior. *Journal of Applied Behavior Analysis, 46*, 1–21.

Blackman, D. (2018). *Operant Conditioning: An Experimental Analysis of Behaviour* (3rd edn). Abingdon: Routledge.

Cooper-Evans, S., Alderman, N., Knight, C. and Oddy, M. (2008). Self-esteem and self-concept as predictors of mood and behaviour during rehabilitation following severe brain injury: An exploratory study. *Neuropsychological Rehabilitation, 18*, 607–626.

Eells, T.D., Kekjelic, E.M. and Lucas, C.P. (1998). What's in a case formulation? *Journal of Psychotherapy Practice and Research, 7*, 144–153.

Freeman, K.A., Anderson, C.M., and Scotti, J.R. (2000). A structured descriptive methodology: Increasing agreement between descriptive and experimental analyses. *Education & Training in Mental Retardation & Developmental Disabilities, 35*, 55–66.

Kelly, G., Todd, J., Simpson, G., Kremer, P. and Martin, C. (2006). The Overt Behaviour Scale (OBS): A tool for measuring challenging behaviours following ABI in community settings. *Brain Injury, 20*, 307–319.

Lerman, D.C. and Iwata, B.A. (1993). Descriptive and experimental analyses of variables maintaining self-injurious behavior. *Journal of Applied Behaviour Analysis, 26*, 293–319.

Lerman, D.C., Iwata, B.A. and Wallace, M.D. (1999). Side effects of extinction: Prevalence of bursting and aggression during the treatment of self-injurious behavior. *Journal of Applied Behavior Analysis, 32*, 1–8.

McGrath, J.C. (2007). *Ethical Practice in Brain Injury Rehabilitation*. New York: Oxford University Press.

O'Neill, R., Horner, R., Albin, R., Sprague, J., Storey, K. and Newton, J. (1997). *Functional Assessment and Program Development for Problem Behavior: A Practical Handbook* (2nd edn). Pacific Grove, CA: Brooks/Cole.

Rahman, B., Alderman, N. and Oliver, C. (2013). The application of a structured descriptive assessment methodology with traumatic brain injury survivors to identify the function of challenging behaviour. *Neuropsychological Rehabilitation: An International Journal, 23*, 501–527.

Tam, S., McKay, A., Sloan, S. and Ponsford, J. (2015). The experience of challenging behaviours following severe TBI: A family perspective. *Brain Injury, 29*, 813–821.

Tate, R. and Perdices, M. (2018). *Single-Case Experimental Designs for Clinical Research and Neurorehabilitation Settings: Planning, Conduct, Analysis and Reporting* (1st edn). Abingdon: Routledge.

Wood, R.Ll. (1987). *Brain Injury Rehabilitation: A Neurobehavioural Approach.* London: Croom Helm.

Wood, R.Ll. and Eames, P. (1981). Application of behaviour modification in the rehabilitation of traumatically brain injured patients. In G. Davey (ed.), *Applications of Conditioning Theory.* London: Methuen.

3 A legal framework for the management of challenging behaviour

Darren Smith and Andrew Worthington

Introduction

The management of challenging behaviour following ABI can only take place within legally defined parameters and changes in legislation have had an increasing impact on the way services and individual professionals operate. In this chapter we review the legal framework and key legislative changes that have come to define the landscape of neurobehavioural services, slow stream rehabilitation and long-term care within an inpatient hospital setting. Whilst the legal aspects are specific to England and Wales, we hope that the issues raised will resonate with a broader readership by providing a detailed insight into this legislative framework and encouraging reflection on how similar issues are managed in other healthcare systems.

Historical background

Neurobehavioural rehabilitation, as distinct from other forms of rehabilitation that catered for physical impairment or emotional and adjustment problems, began to emerge in the 1970s, with increasing realisation of the impact of behavioural and personality changes after ABI (Worthington, Wood, and McMillan, 2017). Prior to the establishment of this speciality, people with disorders of conduct following brain injury were largely excluded from rehabilitation and left to the management of psychiatrists to be treated with 'a supportive calm environment' (Levin, Benton and Grossman, 1982), which often involved sedative medication. Service users often had complicated histories and family dynamics and multiple physical and other co-morbid conditions. The notion of neurobehavioural disability reflected the impact of this complex, pervasive constellation of cognitive-behavioural changes of attention, executive function, diminished insight, poor social judgement, labile mood and problems of impulse control (Wood, 2001). To meet this challenge, neurobehavioural rehabilitation services were organised differently from traditional medical establishments, being neuropsychiatry- or neuropsychology-led with a transdisciplinary team incorporating not only a comprehensive multidisciplinary team of therapists but also rehabilitation assistants (see Chapter 1). They had higher staffing ratios of highly trained and motivated personnel and were costed accordingly.

DOI: 10.4324/9781003083290-4

Over time, multiple reorganisations within the NHS led to a variety of mechanisms for obtaining funding for specialist placements, particularly when 'out of area'. In 1974, around 90 Area Health Authorities were introduced, with responsibility for planning and providing services for their populations. They were in turn replaced by some 200 District Health Authorities in 1982, scattering expertise ever more thinly. The 1989 *Working for Patients* white paper introduced the service-provider split practitioners are familiar with today (subsequently implemented in the National Health Service and Community Care Act in April 1990). This relegated health authorities to the role of buying healthcare from providers and ensured that hospitals and community services would become autonomous trusts with budgets subject to contracts with purchasers.

For the most behaviourally disturbed service users detained under the Mental Health Act (1983) (MHA) funding has tended to be relatively straightforward. Then, as now, neurobehavioural treatment could be bought from specialist centres (known as spot-purchasing), currently through clinical commissioning groups. The legislation specifies certain mandatory processes, which are interwoven with rehabilitation. Service users are subject to care programme approach (CPA) reviews on a six-monthly basis. There is normally a named professional who is contactable, with discharges carefully planned and organised in conjunction with named external professionals.

The healthcare system looked very different 20 years ago. Without a statutory framework to drive admission and treatment, prospects for people being admitted to much-needed rehabilitation on an informal basis were less secure. One health commissioner admitted, 'unless there happens to be an active neurorehabilitation service at a trust within the district, so creating a budget line for a group of patients, most neurorehabilitation purchasing is pragmatically based on individual costs, and uninformed by scientific methods or concern for outcomes' (McCarthy, 1999, p. 298).

Within services there was less oversight from external bodies outside CPA meetings with almost everything managed internally. Safeguarding incidents were not identified as safeguarding in the way they are today, but would been viewed as risk incidents, with only significant incidents being reported out externally. Regardless of admission status, choices were minimal since a services user's care and treatment was still directed and managed by the consultant, although compared to traditional medical services the importance of the wider team in influencing treatment decisions was recognised.

Options for intervention were formulated using outcome measures and observational recording measures, such as the Overt Aggression Scale – Modified for Neurorehabilitation (OAS-MNR) (Alderman, Knight and Morgan, 1997) (see Chapter 5). This scale highlighted the type of behaviour, antecedent and severity of the behaviour, assessing the potential relationship between the environment and behaviour. The data would inform the behaviour support programme, which would target a specific area as described in Chapter 2. This would be led by the consultant psychologist and reviewed in a ward round or team meeting. With team members in agreement about the need for an intervention and the form this would take, a second opinion might be requested to offer an impartial opinion on what was being proposed to further validate the course of action. Following this, the behaviour support plan would be owned and operated by the entire transdisciplinary team (TDT) (see Chapters 6 and 8).

The overall aims of these programmes were to reduce the behaviours to a degree where the person could be reintegrated into the community and either moved home or moved closer to their family. Programmes varied in sophistication, using a variety of the techniques described in Chapter 6, including variants of time-out, differential reinforcement and response-cost. Tangible reinforcers used as part of these interventions varied depending on what motivated service users, such as extra money for additional trips out. Interventions benefitted from an evidence base that testified to their effectiveness when used to manage challenging behaviour expressed by people with ABI. Some of the techniques used in the past, whilst having a clear rationale, demonstrable effectiveness and undertaken with professionalism, would nevertheless be considered less favourably today, including forms of manual handling and the use of aversive stimulation. While the use of seclusion is within the definition of medical treatment in the MHA, it should not be used as part of a treatment plan or in a punitive manner, but as a last resort for the shortest possible time. The legal framework for managing challenging behaviour puts the onus very clearly on the least restrictive practice with the introduction of the Mental Capacity Act (2005), which is discussed below.

Quality and governance

Neurobehavioural services, like others, have also witnessed a steady increase in regulatory oversight and inspection. The Care Quality Commission (CQC) was founded in 2008, replacing the Healthcare Commission, the Commission for Social Care Inspection and the Mental Health Act Commission. Their function was to be responsible for the registration of services, facilitate inspections and monitor health and social care providers under the Health and Social Care Act (2008). Following a planned or unannounced inspection, services receive a rating that can range from Inadequate to Outstanding. There is no set of standards specific for brain injury and CQC ratings are not intended to substitute for measures of clinical or social outcomes.

A further shift in the legislative landscape followed the implementation of the Care Act (2014). This aimed to coalesce disparate areas of legislation for the purpose of protecting vulnerable adults, including (for inpatient services) sections 42–47, which refer to safeguarding responsibilities and the establishment of Safeguarding Adults Boards. Although the focus was on providing clear directions and responsibilities to local authorities rather than clinicians delivering treatment, the legislation has added impetus to measures to embed safeguarding into clinical care.

Detention and deprivation of liberty

The introduction of the Mental Capacity Act (2005) had a major impact on the healthcare system, especially in terms of offering choice and placing individuals with mental capacity in control of their own care and treatment. This can sometimes create uncertainty as to the most appropriate legislation to use in treatment (Richardson, 2010). Previously people who lacked capacity to consent to admission to hospital, but did not overtly object, were treated informally under common law. It was necessary to be a 'patient' under the MHA by reason of mental disorder before the courts could step in and administer matters on a person's behalf. Like most legislation it took time to effect real change at a service level and several years before a person's capacity status really started to have an impact on their care and treatment. For people not formally detained many professionals had implicitly accepted that any deprivation of liberty involved in rehabilitation (and other services) was based on whether a resident was objecting to their care and support or was actively requesting to leave. The courts made clear this was not the case and, in 2007, the Act was amended with the introduction of Deprivation of Liberty Safeguards (DoLS) for adults who lacked capacity and were deprived of their liberty in care homes and hospitals, which included rehabilitation facilities.[1] Further clarification by Supreme Court judgement in the 'Cheshire West' case has set a low bar 'acid test' beyond which additional legal authorisation is required (effectively this is whether the person is subject to continuous supervision and control and whether they are free to leave). This brings the notions of restriction and deprivation of liberty ever closer and has raised concerns about implementation. Within the first year of the acid test being introduced 137,540 applications were submitted (2014–2015) based on the new criteria. This was a significant increase compared to applications made before this hearing 13,700 (2013–2014). These figures continue to rise yearly and have resulted in the framework being not fit for purpose due to local authorities not having adequately trained staff to complete the number of applications being made.

DoLS will be replaced by Liberty Protection Safeguards that were introduced in the Mental Capacity (Amendment) Act (2019), to be applied in domestic settings and requiring a medical assessment of mental disorder, assessment of capacity and a 'necessary and proportionate' assessment to ensure arrangements are appropriate. At the time of writing, their implementation has been delayed.

Mental capacity and supported decision making

Enshrined in the Mental Capacity Act (MCA) is an obligation to ensure all practicable steps are taken to allow a person to exercise capacity, and, in the event that they lack capacity, then decisions must be taken in their best interests using the least restrictive interventions. This raises ethical as well as legal issues, especially in seeking to modify challenging behaviour, some of which may reflect pre-morbid propensities, possibly exacerbated by ABI, and present risks to self and others (see Worthington and Archer, 2009, and Chapter 4 this volume). In practice, professionals have continued to struggle with the implications of mental capacity law in rehabilitation. Severe brain injury and challenging behaviour does not by itself denote lack of capacity; each capacity issue has to be addressed separately, and opinions may differ as to whether or not a person has capacity and, if lacking, what is the least restrictive alternative.

In the case of a person who lacks capacity, professionals may be risk averse, adopting a cautionary principle in acting in what they believe is in the person's best interests (see guidance by Wade and Kitzinger, 2019). The courts have made clear that best interest extends beyond self-interest (see Donnelly, 2009), and professionals should be wary of a 'protection imperative'. A number of judicial observations have been made where cases have come before the courts, which can be helpful for practitioners on the ground. As the judge commented in one case,[2] which may resonate: 'There is a danger ... that the patient is regarded as capable of making a decision that follows medical advice but incapable of one that does not.' In other words, a person consenting to an intervention may not be making a capacitous decision, just as the absence of resistance should not be assumed to indicate informed consent.

The MCA has been criticised for incompatibility with the United Nations Convention on the Rights of Persons with Disabilities (UNCRPD), which the UK ratified in 2009. Although this is beyond the scope of the present chapter, at the heart of these concerns is whether the MCA maintains a narrow medical model of disability in which impairment resides within the person and accepts as an inevitability that there will be some restrictions in a person's life rather than seeing this as in itself something to be challenged (see Clough, 2015). This requires practitioners seeking to address the restrictions associated with challenging behaviour to reconsider the attribution of symptoms and causes of disability. While the role of the brain injury remains central in neurobehavioural rehabilitation, it is not always primary and the relevance of environmental and other contextual factors is always highlighted as being important for causation and for behaviour change.

The impact of legislation over recent years has had a major impact on the way services for challenging behaviour operate and the practice of individuals within those services. This has brought to the fore matters such as consent, risk and best practice, which have always been a central part of neurobehavioural rehabilitation but perhaps not always with the benefit of clear legal parameters. In many ways the care and treatment for service users has been enhanced, although by changing the power dynamics between the professional and recipient of services it has also created different sets of challenges for the professional, which has added another layer of complexity to consider with each intervention, making practice more evidence based. Practice has been improved, with professionals having to justify their actions more than ever.

Inevitably the quantity as well as quality of clinical paperwork and official documentation has increased. Legislation to enhance safeguarding has been ground-breaking in placing adult protection at the forefront of care and treatment, but it comes with an associated bureaucracy for those tasked with the managing, reporting and recording of these processes. The consequences of failing have never been greater, whether this be from a personal or an organisational perspective, with external bodies more involved with service user care than ever before. The increase of external monitoring, legislation and regulation have undoubtedly improved the lives of service users, yet there is a danger that the focus may be shifted to satisfying quality criteria and meeting targets rather than an emphasis on good practice and effectiveness. The ability of regulatory inspection to improve quality has been debated (Smithson et al. 2018; Weenink et al., 2021). Anxiety about the rating a service might achieve can be taxing on managers and clinicians; and the effect of a downward shift in rating can be demoralising. There appears to be no research on the psychological impact for people finding themselves placed in a service that has moved from 'good' to 'inadequate', but one can envisage the stress on families especially if their loved ones are forcibly detained in a service that is deemed to be not fit for purpose.

In the next section we consider some of the many legislative frameworks and legal issues involved in managing challenging behaviour by way of a hypothetical example. For illustrative purposes we focus on a hospital admission for neurobehavioural rehabilitation but many of the same issues arise in community settings.

Case scenario

Pre-admission

To emphasise the personal nature of all such cases we will call our hypothetical service user David. He is a 42-year-old married man with children, who was employed, financially secure and had a large, supportive extended family. David was referred to the service with a hypoxic brain injury caused by cardiac arrest 12 months prior. At the point of the assessment, he was mobile, being fed through a percutaneous endoscopic gastrostomy (PEG, a type of feeding tube) and had complex physical care needs. He also exhibited significant behavioural challenges, which had resulted in several placements being terminated. The long-term goal for David was to be discharged back to the family home following a period of rehabilitation.

All services should have admission criteria, which are based on diagnosis or needs but they should also include treatment potential and the evaluation of presenting risks. A pre-admission assessment including analysis of behavioural evidence ensured that in this case David not only met the clinical criteria for admission but also had the appropriate risk profile. As there is a limit to the type of behaviour that can be safely managed, considerations need to be made in the following areas.

Current resident group

Would David integrate into the current resident group? Would David be a risk to others or vulnerable to retaliation from others?

Environment

Is the environment suitable for David? Is he a security risk? Could he abscond and breach the perimeter, putting himself in danger?

Risk to staff

What is the level of risk towards staff? Is restraint likely to be required? If so, what level of restraint has been needed prior to admission?

Ability to manage behaviours and deliver treatment programmes

Does the service have the expertise to meet David's needs? Can the programmes/treatments required be delivered consistently and safely?

This is basic guidance but is important to get right from the outset. Healthcare is finance driven and a service's inability to safeguard individuals appropriately can result in negative CQC compliance ratings, social media exposure and in some cases criminal charges.

Once the clinical team has made the decision on suitability, the legal basis for David's admission must be ascertained if not already clear. Unless he is being admitted formally for assessment under the auspices of the Mental Health Act, David's capacity to consent to admission needs to be evaluated. Where this is deemed to be lacking it is best practice to request a copy of the best interests decision regarding the transfer, which determined the service was the most appropriate and least restrictive option. Its highly likely these discussions are held informally (especially if in a general hospital) and it can be difficult to obtain the documents, but if admission is challenged further down the line, it is advantageous to have these in situ (for example, Essex County Council vs RF & Ors).

Paying for rehabilitation

Most neurobehavioural rehabilitation in the UK is ultimately paid for by the NHS through local commissioning arrangements. Healthcare funding is a finite resource and there are eligibility criteria to qualify for Continuing Healthcare (CHC) funding, which many people with very challenging behaviour from ABI will meet. Unfortunately, differences between regional criteria, sometimes reflecting local circumstances, can lead to disparities and inequities. In addition, during the course of treatment, any shift from clinical (health) needs to more social needs can trigger a reappraisal of a person's eligibility to healthcare funding, which in turn, depending on the decision, can lead to a complex appeals process. This can be difficult for clinicians to understand and negotiate and families can be bewildered, frustrated and distressed by a lack of funding for their loved one to receive much-needed treatment.

Admission

The assessment phase of rehabilitation starts on Day 1, with the nurses and therapists booking in sessions to start their individual assessments. Assessment of capacity to consent to treatment and consent to share personal information are key areas from a legal perspective, and the outcome of the assessments will provide a clear direction in terms of the need for a legal framework and whom the service can share information with from a family perspective. The latter provides a clear structure for both staff and families as to what information will be communicated to whom. This is key at the start of admission and, if mismanaged, can result in a breach of duty of care or a serious complaint. In the case of David, a clear process was identified following a best interests meeting about the sharing of personal information with his family: all parties were able to agree that his wife would be the main contact and all information would be passed through her.

If David was deemed to meet the criteria for a DoLS, the referral form required for this is Form 1 Standard and Urgent request (ADASS). Prior to making the application the person responsible for making the application should speak to his family to discuss the application, explaining the process, and should gain agreement that a referral should/can be made, establishing that there is no advance decision that could impact on this. Although there are clear timeframes for this, they are rarely met, and confirmation may take many months as a result of some referrals being deemed as low priority. These tend to be low-risk referrals where everyone is in agreement with the placement and treatment. Such referrals could be outstanding for years depending on the local authority's resources (ADASS, 2016).

It can be difficult establishing the identity of the mandated supervisory body; in the UK geographical borders of local authorities vary depending on the postcode, and in some areas supervisory bodies have split regions meaning referrals can be made to the right locality but the incorrect region. A lost or misplaced referral would be a breach of Article 5 of the Human Rights Act (1998), since there would be no procedure prescribed in law supporting the service when it is necessary to deprive a person of their liberty, even though that person lacks capacity to consent to their care and treatment and there is duty to keep them safe.

When completing the DoLS paperwork for David on admission, it would be important to establish what restrictions would be necessary so these can be included within the application. This is often fluid as behaviours can change frequently. Restrictions may be added and removed depending on the level of risk, however there are some key areas/restrictions that professionals should be aware of:

- any enhanced observations (one-to-one)
- locked doors
- restrictive equipment
- medication to control behaviour.

Whilst these assessments are happening, the clinical team also start the process of completing other required mental capacity assessments that should be conducted. David's assessments would be specific to his presentation but in general the following should be considered:

- medication (consider covert medication if required)
- photographs (used on the clinical records)
- PEG/modified diet (unless on normal diet and fluids)
- restrictive equipment (bedrails/hoist and sling/ lap belts or harnesses/tilt and space chairs).

A range of additional mental capacity assessments would be required according to David's clinical needs and behaviours (such as access to the Internet and access to specific visitors) and sometimes in response to local authority specifications or government initiatives. The recent Covid-19 pandemic, for example, resulted in assessments of consent for testing and vaccination, an area that remains contentious today.

Assessment

The initial weeks were about getting to know David, observing and recording his behaviours, establishing what he could do independently and what level of support he required to complete tasks. Assessments by the clinical team would be ongoing until there was enough information to formulate a behaviour support plan (see Chapters 2 and 7). Early on in this process assessment data collected (for example, OAS-MNR). For David this highlighted:

- Verbal aggression: David may shout angrily, make personal insults and swear at staff.
- Physical aggression: David may make threatening gestures towards others or strike others when he is agitated.
- Inappropriate sexual behaviour: He may make inappropriate comments towards female members of staff or attempt to kiss them. He may become tactile with staff, rubbing their arms or legs.
- Wandering: He may wander into areas that are non-communal.

- Inappropriate social behaviour: David may laugh inappropriately, fail to monitor his personal hygiene, excessively apologise or thank a person, invade personal space, and be non-compliant with care tasks.
- Lack of initiation: David may require prompting and supervision for many tasks of daily living.

Other assessment instruments may identify additional behaviours of concern. For example, the Agitated Behaviour Scale, completed by carers, captures their experience of challenging behaviours from working with service users/patients/residents. David was rated as scoring 35/56 which suggested moderate levels of agitation. His frequently occurring behaviours described by carers included:

- short attention span, easy distractibility, inability to concentrate;
- impulsive, impatient, low tolerance for pain or frustration;
- restlessness, pacing, excessive movement;
- pulling at tubes;
- wandering from treatment areas;
- rapid, loud or excessive talking.
- easily initiated crying and/or laughing.

In severe brain injury cases presenting with behaviour disorder, a person's levels of attention, engagement and understanding may preclude formal assessment of cognition, and so structured observations assume great importance. These may be undertaken in joint therapist assessments. For example the speech and language therapist may join a physiotherapy session or occupational therapy session to gain insight into a person's communication through a range of functional situations. In David's case these highlighted widespread impairments, especially affecting memory, attention, language and information processing, which affected most aspects of his daily living. As a result, he would require enhanced one-to-one support throughout the day.

Safeguarding

As identified above, the notion of safeguarding has transformed the way neurobehavioural services and others now operate. It is set out in some detail below. Safeguarding vulnerable adults is a key requirement for any service and regulatory body, with 'safe' being one of the CQC's 'fundamental standards' (Care Quality Commission, 2023). However, due to different safeguarding criteria, there is a lack of consistency among professionals and between local authorities about what constitutes a reportable safeguarding incident. It is important to rehabilitation professionals to establish clear links with their local safeguarding team and gain an understanding of what they deem to be safeguarding. This information can usually be found on a local authority's website and some areas now publish a matrix of what they interpret as reportable incidents and non-reportable incidents. Understanding and applying a matrix of safeguarding incidents demonstrates compliance with the local authority's arrangements. It also provides evidence of decision making if questioned. For example, if the CQC or a local quality monitoring body deem an incident to be reportable during an inspection even though it may not meet a local authority criterion. Failing to report incidents or evidencing the decision could result in a negative CQC grading such as 'inadequate' or 'requires improvement' and bring about more frequent inspections. In a worst-case scenario the service could be prosecuted directly under the CQC's enforcement policy that was introduced in 2015.

Every site should strive to be transparent in relation to safeguarding; and all services will undoubtedly have incidents at some stage that require a safeguarding notification. It is best practice to have a clear dialogue and, where possible, inviting the local safeguarding team to a meeting on site on a regular basis is certainly beneficial. This enables clear communication around reportable incidents and non-reportable incidents on site. It also provides clear evidence that all incidents are discussed with the local authority during inspections.

Applying matrix criteria is essential in ensuring that a service remains transparent and maintains a balance between not over-reporting nor diluting the actual process. For illustration, if David's verbal aggression was found to be directed towards a specific peer this would likely be seen as risk behaviour and recorded on the OAS-MNR. This could be documented as non-reportable safeguarding and monitored, so, if further incidents between David and his peer occurred, it could be escalated to a full notification on the basis of an identified a pattern of behaviour or trend.

In David's case, three separate incidents were recorded towards the same peer in a month. The first two were documented internally, following the guidance of the local authority matrix; the third incident was reported out externally since there was a clear pattern. Prior to making the safeguarding notification, it is best practice to assess capacity to establish if the 'adult at risk' can consent to the referral and being part of the safeguarding process. In this example, the adult at risk would be the peer whom David was targeting. Some service users will have capacity in this area and may decline, stating they do not wish the referral to be made. The clinical team can override their wishes if they believe or have evidence that:

- it is in the public interest;
- there is the risk of serious harm;
- there is a risk of serious crime, or a serious crime is suspected;
- the ability of the adult at risk to consent is affected by threatening behaviour;
- seeking consent would increase risks to the adult at risk or others;
- there is a risk of the service user potentially being unduly influenced or coerced by another person.

With regard to David, his peer lacked capacity, so a best interests decision was made by the clinical team and the family. It is important that the family are part of the decision-making process, understand the circumstances around the incident/s, and can advocate on the service user's behalf. This is key when evidencing that you are applying the safeguarding personal process, showing the process to be person-centred and outcome-focused rather than simply a clinically-led process.

Once the safeguarding notification has been submitted, a CQC notification then needs to be completed (abuse or allegations of abuse concerning a person who uses the service), and contact made with the commissioners for both parties. This is easier to achieve in hospital settings due to a likely funding commissioning contact or an attached care coordinator. By contrast, in a care home or residential service, notification tends to be made to the duty clinician at the health funding agency or with social services.

The type of notification triggered by David's behaviour would normally be closed with no further action, since there was no harm caused and staff de-escalated the situation. Further information may be requested to satisfy the local safeguarding team. If assurances are not provided this incident could result in the incident being deemed as an s42 enquiry (Care Act 2014), which means a full investigation and subsequent report would be required. In most cases the s42 enquiry would be allocated to the service to complete, however in more complex cases the safeguarding team may allocate themselves and visit the service for a full review.

Raising a safeguarding notification with the local authority should never be seen as negative. The process is aimed to be supportive and can be used to a service's own benefit. A professional raising a safeguarding concern with the local authority based on the fact a resident is at risk of abuse (even though no abuse has observed at the time), provides an opportunity to highlight specific concerns that, if not addressed, would ultimately lead a to serious safeguarding event. The concern could be based on something outside the professional's own control, such as a hospital intervention or the involvement of an external party in a self-neglect case, posing a risk of general hospital admission in the future. Clinicians and managers should note that taking the time to complete referrals for self-neglect is best practice but also defensible practice, since a general hospital is very likely to make an immediate safeguarding referral against the service for neglect. As such, making the local authority aware of issues first prevents the concern escalating to a full s42 enquiry.

Rehabilitation

As the clinical team complete their assessments, these will be formally shared and discussed to understand the goals and management plans of each professional, or agree joint plans when rehabilitation is provided by a TDT. In David's case, the outcome of the assessments resulted in the following being recommended:

- clear guidance on the best way to communicate;
- one-to-one enhanced support;
- errorless learning orientation programme;

- positive behavioural support plan;
- response-cost programme aimed at inappropriate sexual behaviour;
- toileting programme;
- structured hygiene programme – including facilitation.

With goals agreed, professionals can review areas that are required to be supported by a mental capacity assessment and where necessary a best interests decision. The DoLS referral can then be updated as additional restrictions may be needed. For David, the restrictive interventions likely to need review would be the one-to-one enhanced support, the response-cost programme and the structured hygiene programme since the rest of the proposed interventions are not restrictive.

On completion of the required mental capacity assessments, a best interests meeting should be held as soon as possible to avoid any delay in the planned interventions. Family involvement is important, and some best interests meetings can be held over the telephone, but for more complex matters it is advisable, where possible, to call a family meeting to discuss the planned interventions and what the clinical team hope to achieve. It is highly recommended that the commissioners who fund the treatment are invited to attend this meeting, since additional funding would be required for one-to-one enhanced support should it prove necessary.

Once the best interests decision and the agreed plans for intervention are in place, the original DoLS that was submitted on admission may need to be amended to include the above. Procedures vary between regions and some areas have online forms, whilst others require the ADASS forms to be completed and sent to them. It is recommended that services make contact directly with the relevant local authority DoLS team to establish how they would like to be notified.

Discharge

Establishing admission goals at the outset, even if these have to be adapted during the rehabilitation process, should also anticipate the likely timing and conditions for discharge.

This may involve a return to the family home as, in David's case, a step down to a less secure rehabilitative setting or a move to a longer-term place of residence for people unable to return to their former home. Capacity to make decisions regarding place of residence on discharge should be specifically assessed, evidence showing that cognitive status as measured by psychometric tests is a poor predictor (Mackenzie, Lincoln and Newby, 2008). Experience shows that such transitions can be very difficult to get right, occurring too soon (through self-discharge or lack of funding), too late or too slowly. Around the time of admission, a conversation should be held with families explaining that funding is limited and will be reviewed. They should be informed that following a CHC assessment they may be served 28 days' notice if the criteria are not met, in addition to the fact that Social Services may not get involved immediately if that were to occur, and that care responsibility may be left with the family in the event of a hiatus. Communication delays between health and social care are not unusual. Worthington and Oldham (2006) reported that discharge delays were especially likely for people who had additional medical needs that would need to be managed in the community and for people for whom funding responsibility was at least in part shifted from health to social care.

Conclusion

This chapter has highlighted how changes to legislation have affected and changed professional practice, acknowledging that the processes are not controlled by clinicians, nor can clinical decisions be made in the way they have been in the past. Making decisions about how best to respond to challenging behaviour in ABI rehabilitation is a complex endeavour that involves legal and ethical as well as clinical considerations. There is now a greater need to engage with the service user who, if they have capacity, can make their own decisions; or, if they lack capacity, to engage with the family and reach a joint decision based on the individual's best interests. The case scenario of David is a typical admission within neurobehavioural services that illustrates the variety of legal frameworks that are applicable before, during and throughout admission and in readiness for discharge. Professionals may express frustration and feel they should have the primacy in clinical decision making. Yet rehabilitation is rarely about purely clinical decisions and is too important to be left solely to medical or other healthcare professionals. Legislation provides a framework to ensure vulnerable people are protected from abuse and malpractice but, even in this regard, it can fall short. Familiarity with the parameters of professional practice laid down by legislation, however, should ensure that rehabilitation services and individual healthcare professionals work to ensure that legislation works *for* them rather than *against* them; and where there are inevitable tensions, these can be highlighted and resolved within the law so that the services and healthcare professionals can withstand any criticism if put to the test before the courts.

Notes

1 See *HL v United Kingdom* 45508/999 [2004] ECHR 471.
2 *Heart of England NHS Foundation Trust v JB* [2014] EWCOP 342 [27–28].

Further reading

Department of Health and Social Care (2022). National framework for NHS continuing healthcare and NHS-funded nursing care. https://www.gov.uk/government/publica tions/national-framework-for-nhs-continuing-healthcare-and-nhs-funded-nursing-care#full-publication-update-history [accessed: 13.02.2023].

Keene, R.K. (2019). DoLS, the backlog and the consequences – the LGO reports. https://www.mentalcapacitylawandpolicy.org.uk/dols-the-backlog-and-the-consequences-the-lgo-reports/ [accessed: 13.02.2023].Mental Health Act 2007, c.12. https://www.legislation.gov.uk/ukpga/2007/12/contents [accessed: 13.02.2023].

National Health Service (2022). Care programme approach. https://www.england.nhs.uk/wp-content/uploads/2021/07/B0526-care-programme-approach-position-statement-v2.pdf [accessed: 13.02.2023].

Norfolk Safeguarding Adults Board (2021). Safeguarding adults review: Joanna, Jon and Ben.https://www.norfolksafeguardingadultsboard.info/assets/SARs/SAR-Joanna-Jon-and-Ben/SAR-Rpt-Joanna-JonBen_FINAL-PUBLICATION02-June2021.pdf [accessed: 13.02.2023].

Samuel, M. (2020). Continuing healthcare assessments resume following covid suspension with backlog of 25,000 to clear. https://www.communitycare.co.uk/2020/08/25/continuing-healthcare-assessments-resume-following-covid-suspension-backlog-25000-clear/ [accessed: 13.02.2023].

Wilson, J. (2023). Mental health law online: Annual review 2022. https://www.mentalhealthlaw.co.uk/Cheshire_West_and_Chester_Council_v_P_(2014)_UKSC_19 [accessed: 13.02.2023].

References

ADASS (2016). Advice note for managing and processing cases generated by the Supreme Court decision in 2014 in relation to deprivation of liberty safeguards. https://www.adass.org.uk/media/5297/additional-dols-safeguards-final.pdf [accessed: 13.02.2023].

Alderman, N., Knight, C., and Morgan, C. (1997). Use of a modified version of the Overt Aggression Scale in the measurement and assessment of aggressive behaviours following brain injury. *Brain Injury*, *11* (7), 503–523.

Care Act (2014), c.23. https://www.legislation.gov.uk/ukpga/2014/23/contents/enacted [accessed: 13.02.2023].

Care Quality Commission (2023). *The Fundamental Standards*. https://www.cqc.org.uk/about-us/fundamental-standards [accessed: 13.02.2023].

Clough, B. (2015). 'People like that': Realising the social model in mental capacity jurisprudence. *Medical Law Review*, *23* (1), 53–80.

Donnelly, M. (2009). Best interests, patient participation and the Mental Capacity Act 2005. *Medical Law Review*, *17* (1), 1–29.

Essex Chambers (2015). *Essex County Council v RF & Ors*. https://www.39essex.com/information-hub/case/essex-county-council-v-rf-ors [accessed: 13.02.2023].

Health and Social Care Act (2008), c.14. https://www.legislation.gov.uk/ukpga/2008/14/contents [accessed: 13.02.2023].

Human Rights Act 1998, c.42. https://www.legislation.gov.uk/ukpga/1998/42/contents [accessed: 13.02.2023].

Levin, H.S., Benton, A.L. and Grossman, R.G. (1982). *Neurobehavioral Consequences of Closed Head Injury*. New York: Oxford University Press.

Mackenzie, J.A., Lincoln, N.B., and Newby, G.J. (2008). Capacity to make a decision about discharge destination after stroke: A pilot study. *Clinical Rehabilitation*, *22* (12), 1116–1126.

McCarthy, M. (1999). Purchasing neurorehabilitation in the UK National Health Service. *Neuropsychological Rehabilitation*, 9 (3–4), 295–303.

Mental Capacity Act (2005), c.9. https://www.legislation.gov.uk/ukpga/2005/9/contents [accessed: 13.02.2023].

Richardson, G. (2010). Mental capacity at the margin: The interface between two acts. *Medical Law Review*, *18*, 1–22.

Smithson, R., Richardson, E., Roberts, J., Walshe, K., Wenzel, L., Robertson, R., Boyd, A., Allen, T. and Proudlove, N. (2018). *Impact of Care Quality Commission on Provider Performance: Room for Improvement.* Manchester: The Kings Fund/Manchester Business School.

Wade, D.T. and Kitzinger, C. (2019). Making healthcare decisions in a person's best interests when they lack capacity: Clinical guidance based on a review of evidence. *Clinical Rehabilitation*, *33* (10), 1571–1585.

Weenink, J.W., Wallenburg, I., Leistikow, I. and Bal, R.A. (2021). Publication of inspection frameworks: A qualitative study exploring the impact on quality improvement and regulation in three healthcare settings. *BMJ Quality & Safety*, *30* (10), 804–811.

Wood, R.Ll. (2001). Understanding neurobehavioural disability. In Wood, R.Ll. and McMillan, T.M. (eds). *Neurobehavioural Disability and Social Handicap Following Traumatic Brain Injury*. Hove: Psychology Press, pp. 3–27.

Worthington, A. and Archer, N. (2009). Assessment and management of risk. In M. Oddy and A. Worthington (eds). *Rehabilitation of Executive Disorders Following Brain Injury*. Oxford, Oxford University Press, pp. 299–326.

Worthington, A.D. and Oldham, J.B. (2006). Delayed discharge from rehabilitation after brain injury. *Clinical Rehabilitation*, *20* (1), 79–82.

Worthington, A., Wood, R.Ll. and McMillan, T. (2017). Neurobehavioural disability over the past four decades. In T. McMillan and R. Ll. Wood (eds). *Neurobehavioural Disability and Social Handicap Following Traumatic Brain Injury* (2nd edn). Abingdon: Psychology Press, pp. 3–29.

Section II

Assessment and formulation

General principles and methods

4 Assessment of behavioural risk in acquired brain injury

Paul Mooney

Introduction

Acquired brain injury (ABI) has been linked with psychiatric morbidity (Carroll et al., 2014) as well as behavioural disturbance, including criminality (Williams et al., 2018). Studies have shown a higher prevalence of criminal and delinquent behaviour in those with ABI compared to non-ABI cohorts (Katzin, Andine, Hofvander, Billstedt and Wallinus, 2020; Carswell et al., 2004; Hux et al., 1998). Those with ABI have also been cited to exhibit increased levels of aggression, linked with poor social functioning, as well as a range of other clinically relevant factors (Vaishnavi, Rao and Fann, 2009). Indeed, the acquisition of a brain injury can also influence the development of numerous clinical problems that may lead to reduced regulatory ability and increased behavioural disturbance, including sleep disorders (Gerald et al., 2022), anxiety disorders (Mallya et al., 2015) and new-onset major depression (Vaishnavi, Rao and Fann, 2009).

Every survivor of ABI will have their own unique experience and recovery journey, dependent on the area and severity of damage endured, and type and quality of support provided to them; as such, the development of antisocial or criminal behaviour is not necessarily, an outcome of ABI. The orbitofrontal cortex has been suggested to be related to the development of antisocial behaviour (Morgan and Lilienfeld, 2000) and dysfunction of the temporal lobe (Tonkonogy, 1991) and prefrontal cortex (Siever, 2008) have also been implicated in the manifestation of violence and aggression, including the manifestation of temporo-limbic disorders. With such a wide array of experience and of outcomes of ABI, it can therefore be challenging to predict acts of violence and aggression, sexual disinhibition or offending, or other acts of antisocial behaviour in this population.

In many areas of applied psychology, such as clinical and forensic, behavioural risk and its assessment have been a focus of research for decades. The term 'behavioural risk' is used in this context to describe a wide range of challenging and/or offending behaviours that may arise as the result of ABI, including interpersonal violence, self-harm, property damage, fire-setting and sexually inappropriate behaviours (Mooney and Alderman, 2022). Over the

DOI: 10.4324/9781003083290-6

years, clinicians and academics alike have attempted better to understand and formulate behaviour disorders and hence reduce re-offending. However, there has been limited research on risk assessment in the field of brain injury, despite acknowledgement that the frequency and intensity of challenging behaviours in this complex population can be of clinical significance (Rao et al., 2009).

Risk assessment in clinical and forensic populations

Historically, risk assessment for violence and sexual offending has included a range of methodologies, such as clinical judgement, actuarial and dynamic assessment and structured professional judgement.

Prior to the development of any structured methods for the assessment of risk, a clinician's own professional judgement was typically relied upon in courts and in clinical practice to determine the level of risk a person presents. However, the seminal paper by Ennis and Litwack (1974) highlighted the fallibility of clinical judgement, citing it to be like 'flipping coins in the courtroom'. As such, clinical judgement, even that of experienced clinicians, was deemed to be no more accurate than chance, and while of course clinical judgement is still used in daily clinical practice to manage risk and behaviour, it is arguably less favourable than other, more scientific approaches.

Subsequently, efforts were focused on developing quantifiable methods, with the introduction of actuarial (or 'static') measures such as the Violence Risk Appraisal Guide (VRAG; Harris, Rice and Quinsey, 1993), Static-99 (Hanson, 1997) and the Risk Matrix 2000 (Thornton et al., 2003; Thornton 2010). While there was initial promise, such tools lacked sensitivity to behavioural change as a result of treatment. As such, a person was unable to reduce their level of risk scored on these measures, as they were based solely on historical and therefore unchangeable factors. Another weakness was that the tools were validated only for specific populations, primarily prison and forensic mental health services, with research indicating their lack of reliability and validity in other populations, such as learning disability and autism (Lindsay et al., 2008). At the time of writing, there is little research that has been conducted with consideration to the ABI population, although clinical logic would indicate that many participants in forensic mental health validation samples would be likely to have suffered some form of ABI, judging by the nature of their offending behaviour and maladaptive lifestyles. The degree to which these samples have included participants who exhibited pre-morbid offending behaviour vs post-brain injury has not been explored in validation studies.

Research has also considered dynamic factors that may be predictive of violence risk in forensic mental health, with some studies focusing on psychiatric diagnoses, such as personality disorder (Hodgins and Riaz, 2011), specific symptoms (Watts et al., 2003), use of substances (Hodgins, 2011), and presence of affective symptoms (Beaudoin et al., 2019). The Short-Term Assessment of Risk and Treatability (START; Nicholls et al., 2007), was designed as a dynamic measure of risk, and provides 20 items that have been empirically linked to the commission of violent behaviour, including substance use, mental state, social skills, rule adherence and insight. Research has shown that in forensic populations, the tool is predictive of multiple risk outcomes, including violence (Marriott et al., 2017).

Structured professional judgement (SPJ) tools, such as the Historical Clinical Risk-20 (HCR-20) violence risk assessment (Webster et al., 1995), Sexual Violence Risk-20 (SVR-20) assessment (Boer et al., 1997), and other later tools such as the Risk of Sexual Violence Protocol (RSVP; Hart, Kropp and Laws, 2003), have arguably become the most commonly used methods of risk assessment in forensic populations. However, despite a number of studies highlighting their benefits, the validity of such measures has been criticised (Tully, 2017), and clinicians can find the measures time consuming, with one professional often being tasked to complete them rather than a team. This could limit the reliability and validity of a given assessment.

Given that SPJ measures were not designed to consider the influence of ABI on challenging behaviour, they may be unsuitable for ABI populations, as they arguably lack sensitivity and specificity to the complexities of the ABI population. Research by Alderman, Major and Brooks (2018), for example, has indicated that the START lacked predictive accuracy for risk of aggression and violence in their sample. This is not to say that these tools do not have a place in clinical practice with ABI, as they can be helpful aide memoires for clinicians dealing with challenging forensic issues, but caution should be exercised when reporting their outcomes and methodological robustness in any form of judicial situation.

The presence of a brain injury presents significant challenges in the assessment of risk, especially given the diversity of causes of neurological damage and ways in which it can impact on decision making, impulse control, anxiety and a range of other clinically relevant variables. Existing forensic risk assessment tools have, to date, lacked validity and reliability for the ABI population, and the variables often explored by such schemes may either be of limited scope (perhaps only reflecting pre-morbid behaviour and personality) or be outweighed by the nature of a person's neurological damage and the unique impact it may have had on their life.

SPJs beyond forensic mental health

As previously stated, there has been a relative paucity of research seeking to validate SPJ measures in populations outside of male forensic mental health populations. However, work in neurodevelopmental pathways (that is, learning disability and autism populations) has suggested that both actuarial and SPJ measures of risk may be of limited utility. In a study of 212 offenders with learning disability and autism (Lindsay et al., 2008), it was found that actuarial tools were unsuccessful in predicting risk of aggression towards others and self in a 6-month and 12-month period. This is perhaps unsurprising as actuarial measures contain numerous items relating to formal charges and convictions, which people with learning disability or autism tend to avoid, instead being directed to obtain support in community or residential therapeutic settings. In addition, this research found that the HCR-20 was predictive of violence during the review period, but that its predictive accuracy was less acute than for mainstream populations. It was also less predictive than dynamic measures such as the Emotional Problems Scale (EPS; Prout and Strohmer, 1991), which was originally designed as a way of determining treatment needs and measuring outcomes across 12 domains of functioning, rather than as a risk assessment. It is also worth noting that the participants in such studies tend to have forensic histories, and are placed in secure hospitals or locked services or they access community forensic teams. The extent to which the HCR-20 would be suitable for non-forensic learning disability and autism clients who exhibit challenging behaviour remains unclear. In addition, such research also has typically focused on those with mild to borderline learning disability/autism, and not those with moderate or severe forms of these diagnoses; as such, the ability to generalise the results to the population as a whole may be limited.

Clinical practice in ABI and neurodevelopmental services tends to focus on the importance of a functional assessment to determine behavioural function, as a priority over the use of forensic risk assessments, much like in ABI services. Arguably, functional assessment can, and perhaps should, also be used as a means of assessing risk, as many psychologists have found that one of the most powerful predictors of future behaviour tends to be past behaviour (Webb and Sheeran, 2006; Wood, Quinn and Kashy, 2002).

The majority of research into SPJ tools has focused on male perpetrators of violence, and studies into the use of HCR-20, for example, have suggested that it may be more helpful in assessing men than women (Garcia-Mansilla, Rosenfeld and Cruise, 2011). Research by de Vogel et al. (2012) added that the HCR-20 was useful when assessing women, but that it required the addition of items that the authors named the 'Female Additional Manual' (FAM), comprising items that they suggested were specific to female experience, including pregnancy at a young age, parenting difficulties, suicidal behaviour/self-harm and prostitution. Subsequent research has indicated that the addition of the FAM for this population (de Vogel, Bruggeman and Lancel, 2019) aided risk prediction.

Cultural factors have been cited as important to consider in the application of risk assessment tools. Shepherd and Lewis-Fernandez (2016), for example, reported on the 2015 ruling by a Canadian court (*Ewart vs Canada*) that several risk instruments, including the VRAG, Static-99 and others, were inadequate for use with Aboriginal prisoners, due to the inadequate evidence base for the population as well as being susceptible to cultural biases. There remains. however, a lack of research on the impact of culture on other SPJ risk measures and guidance around their adaptation and application in a variety of populations.

It is clear that, despite a great deal of empirical research over the past 40 years, there remains much to understand about the process of risk assessment and prediction even in mental health populations, let alone for ABI, neurodevelopmental and other important, and often overlooked, clinical populations.

Challenging behaviour in ABI

People with an acquired brain injury, and in particular those requiring neurobehavioural rehabilitation (NbR), have been the focus of a growing literature over the past 40 years. Research has identified the benefits of the use of behavioural and social interventions as well as the use of structured environments and a transdisciplinary team in the reduction of behavioural disturbance. Furthermore, the use of observational tools such as the OAS-MNR (Alderman, Knight and Morgan, 1997) has been cited as central in the development of our understanding of the functions and antecedents to challenging behaviour. As such, it may be the case that, in line with early behavioural research, the most efficient predictor of future behaviour may be past behaviour, although this view of course does not take into consideration the impact of therapeutic interventions designed to alleviate risk.

There has been little by way of research into how clinicians, or teams, can best conceptualise and assess the risk of people with brain injury and challenging behaviour in these settings, beyond the use of behavioural tools such as the OAS-MNR. The prevailing view, however, is that existing SPJ tools may be helpful in specific clinical cases but may not be the best choice of assessment if requiring a service-wide solution. It is clear that more research is required in this area to ensure mitigation of risk to the patient and staff supporting them (Alderman, Major and Brooks, 2018).

Proposing a risk assessment framework for neurological services

Typically, patients in forensic mental health and prison services are subject to a risk assessment on a regular basis, most often the HCR-20 and/or START. This is reviewed regularly. It considers the patient's risk of violence, self-harm, suicide and damage to property, among other areas of behavioural disturbance. These assessments aim to underpin the development and review of care and treatment plans that help the patient to contain their risks while also providing appropriate intervention, although clinical experience has suggested that some clinicians may feel they are a paper exercise, especially when they are time poor. For neurological and neurobehavioural services, the evidence base does not currently support the use of such tools; however, it would make sense to utilise a structured approach to the assessment, with factors that are unique to the brain injury population being considered.

The process of conducting violence risk assessments tend to follow a common path, regardless of the tool used: formal assessment, including a review of the most salient factors that influence risk; consideration of risk scenarios, where situations are outlined in which the person's risk may escalate; and development of a risk management plan, where a team considers what support and interventions might mitigate the identified risk(s) within a given time period. Such a clear and rational line of thinking should be adopted, with some alterations and guidance, for a neurobehavioural population.

Considerations in neurobehavioural risk assessment

Before considering how risk should be assessed in neurobehavioural services, we must first be clear regarding the aims of assessment, and the philosophy underlying the process.

The first consideration is that staff training is paramount to any robust risk assessment and management system. All staff working within a given service should receive sufficient training to understand the nature and form of risk, specifically violence and aggression, self-harming, suicide and other forms of behavioural disturbance, where required. A shared understanding as to the common functions of such behaviours, and the team's clinical approach to them, is intrinsic to the success of any service and to obtain positive outcomes for patients.

The second consideration is that risk assessment should be viewed as a *team* activity, and not the responsibility of one person or profession. The whole team should value the process of risk assessment, as this helps keep individuals (including the patient) safe, otherwise there is a risk of a breakdown in the process, which can lead to poor outcomes. Typically, neurobehavioural rehabilitation services are advised to be delivered using a 'transdisciplinary team' approach (Alderman, 2003), where clinicians aim to come together to provide holistic and transformative solutions to behavioural problems, and so the collective skills of a team should be seen to be central in the assessment and management of risk.

The third consideration is that any risk assessment should be viewed in the same manner as a clinical formulation, and they should be in a state of continual revision and refinement (Antaki, Barnes and Leudar, 2005). As such, risk assessments should be reviewed regularly, and, while it may take time for some identified variables to change in this population (and indeed, some may remain static), there must remain the understanding that behavioural change is possible and is a core outcome in rehabilitation. The frequency of review may be mediated by the policies inherent within a given organisation, but should be on a monthly basis, or less should there be a significant incident or emergence of a new maladaptive behaviour.

Finally, a clear case conceptualisation and formulation should be available, alongside a robust functional behaviour analysis that uses validated observational tools to collect behavioural data (for example, OAS-MNR; Alderman, Knight and Morgan, 1997). Responsibility for the completion of these tools should be shared, following the transdisciplinary approach.

The process of neurobehavioural risk assessment

Given the long and, at times chequered, history of risk assessment in forensic services, it is important to ensure that any NbR risk assessment is (i) fit for purpose for the individual, (ii) fit for purpose as regards the general population in question, and (iii) is dynamic in nature, allowing a team's understanding of a person and that their disability will change over time as interventions are implemented and hopefully successful.

The process of NbR risk assessment follows the logic already adhered to by forensic tools such as the HCR-20, whereby teams identify those factors increasing risk, identify and outline the situations in which risk is present, and finally formulate a plan to mitigate and treat these risks. Below is a suggested process specific to working with patients in neurobehavioural rehabilitation services; it comprises a number of key areas that should be synthesised into a clinical formulation of risk.

Assessment

Pre-morbid personality and behaviour

Studies have indicated that pre-morbid personality traits and behaviour may be exacerbated in individuals with acquired brain injury (Norup and Mortensen, 2015). As such, developing an understanding of the person's life and presentation prior to the brain injury will be important in understanding potential behavioural, relational and emotional problems outlined in the formulation.

Symptom analysis

The specific issues relating to the individual's brain injury will be an important aspect of the assessment. As such, teams should consider the specific areas of localised damage, which may yield hypotheses regarding intervention and prognosis, as well as currently displayed symptoms or deficits known to have occurred as a result of the brain injury. Examples may include impaired decision making, increased anxiety and stress (exacerbated by the loss of functional abilities, for example), or indeed a myriad of cognitive impairments that may require tailored intervention.

Type/frequency/intensity of challenging behaviour

The use of tools such as the OAS-MNR (Alderman, Knight and Morgan, 1997) is advocated as a means of recording accurate behavioural data that provide teams with an insight into the type, frequency and intensity of the behaviour, as well as identifying antecedents and other important variables. As such, the formulation benefits from a rich overview of the current presentation and variables that may influence behaviour.

Protective factors

Historically, forensic risk assessments lacked focus or inclusion of protective factors that would aid a person's resilience and mitigate risk. However, since the turn of the millennium, risk assessment has slowly started to integrate this vital area, with inclusion in SPJ tools, such as the START, and published theories such as the Good Lives Model (GLM) (Ward, 2002), which aimed to identify and develop the domains of an offender's life that provided meaning and value. For NbR patients, it is vital that there is focus placed upon any factors that may aid their resilience and ability both to manage stress and to maintain motivation through treatment and adversity. The use of models such as PERMA (Seligman, 2011), which considers factors that contribute to the well-being and quality of life of an individual (for example, experiencing Positive Emotion, Engagement, Relationships, Meaning and Accomplishments), may help teams and patients to identify such factors and ultimately to maintain hope for their future.

Formulation synthesis

Being able to synthesise the above data into a clear formulation of a patient's risk can be challenging, especially where teams are faced with a multitude of data sources or, as the case can be, a lack of them. To aid this synthesis, a conceptual model should be used that provides an overarching structure and focus. Any theoretical model can be used to meet this need, one such being the 5Ps (Johnstone and Dallos, 2014) which posits five core areas of consideration (presenting problem, predisposing, precipitating, perpetuating and protective factors). Such models are widely used across a variety of service types, and so are not only familiar to clinicians, but accessible for various staff and patients. Using such a model is generally seen as good practice and it is a helpful way of collating information in a methodical way with a team.

The team formulation of these data should culminate in a general agreement as to the level of risk presented by the patient across the key domains of risk (for example, violence, self-harm, suicide, damage to property, sexual). While some may view labelling a risk as low, moderate or high as arbitrary, it should help the team to formally prioritise domains of need.

Functional assessment

Patients in NbR services would benefit from functional assessment, which seeks to identify the functions of a given challenging behaviour via a thorough review of behavioural data. Such behavioural data are often collated through observational tools (for example, OAS-MNR), psychometric tests (for example, Motivation Assessment Scale; Durrand and Crimmins, 1988) and official incident reports, and they help to refine hypotheses as to the underlying function of behaviour. These hypotheses are often summarised as to obtain social attention or something tangible, to escape or avoid an aversive stimulus, or to meet sensory needs.

Management and treatment planning

This part of the process aims to draw together the team's understanding of what strategies might reduce the patient's risk in the coming review period. As a starting point, it can be helpful to consider therapy-interfering behaviours (that is, those behaviours that may inhibit a patient's engagement in treatment, such as poor motivation, lack of insight or 'acting up' in group sessions), as well as therapy-interfering limitations (that is, cognitive deficits that might influence the patient's ability to recall and/or use information, to maintain concentration or to use social problem solving). Without such consideration, treatment efficacy may be limited. Next, teams may find it useful to refer to other data sources that may be used for clinical purposes, which not only provide another, rich source of information, but also aid in ensuring the assessment is data-led. For example, many neurological services use tools such as the SAS-NOS (Alderman, Wood and Williams, 2011), which has been shown to be a reliable and valid measure of outcomes across a number of domains for this population. In addition, a tentative relationship between SASNOS and risk has been suggested by Alderman, Major and Brooks (2018). The review of such data can help teams to further refine the areas of concern for a particular case.

Practical application of the risk assessment process

The proposed ABI risk assessment process is based upon the understanding that the relevant data collection in the form of background history, observations and outcome measures that should be consulted, have already been completed, at least in part, in order to fully assess a patient's risk. As such, services should ensure that there is a culture of 'data collection', where staff have received training and guidance on the application and efficacy of behavioural measures (such as OAS-MNR) and clinical measures (such as SASNOS). Ensuring a feedback loop about the data generated from these is also vital, to ensure that staff see and understand the results of the assessments that they have spent time completing. Such a culture is arguably more receptive to the process of reflection and formulation.

At times, risk assessment can feel laborious to some busy clinicians; a paper exercise to satisfy an unknown, or perhaps misunderstood, need. However, in neurobehavioural services, a transdisciplinary risk assessment process should be seen as integral to ensuring the safety of patients and staff and promoting a culture of reflection and empathy towards those we treat – and each other. Given that traditional risk measures used in forensic mental health services are likely to be inefficient and inadequate for this challenging and heterogeneous population, adherence to a logical and robust (yet flexible) process is important in ensuring a scientific approach to risk assessment and management.

As a final point of reflection, the term 'risk assessment' is a loaded one; it automatically focuses our attention on the negative (that is, the risk itself) and, as a result, many clinicians and teams can forget to balance this with a focus on the protective factors that may aid resilience. In addition, characteristics that may emerge or be exacerbated as a result of ABI, such as impaired insight and decision making, run the risk of being viewed as pathological, with interventions seeking to eradicate these. However, increasingly, clinicians are seeking to reframe how they work with such characteristics, with consideration as to how to understand their function and support the client to meet their needs in more pro-social or adaptive ways. Perhaps across all service types, there still remains the need to reframe our clinical view, and to change the narrative from assessing risk to assessing needs and strengths, with greater focus on understanding what has happened to the person (rather than considering what they have done wrong), following the Power Threat Meaning Framework (PTMF; Johnstone and Boyle, 2018). The PTMF was developed as a response to criticisms of the limiting nature of psychiatric diagnosis and it provides an alternative way of conceptualising a person's problems by supporting understanding of the unique contexts of behaviour and supporting consideration of how a person has survived in a non-judgemental manner. This fundamental shift, moving away from a purely risk-oriented approach and towards a more evidence-based and positive rehabilitation approach, highlights the critical need for formulation to play a central role in guiding the often-complex therapeutic work in neurobehavioural rehabilitation services.

References

Alderman, N. (2003). Rehabilitation of behaviour disorders. In B.A. Wilson (ed.), *Neuropsychological Rehabilitation: Theory and Practice*. Hove: Psychology Press.

Alderman, N., Knight, C. and Morgan, C. (1997). Use of a modified Overt Aggression Scale in the measurement and assessment of aggressive behaviours following brain injury. *Brain Injury, 11* (7), 503–523.

Alderman, N., Major, G. and Brooks, J. (2018). What can structured professional judgement tools contribute to management of neurobehavioural disability? Predictive validity of the Short-Term Assessment of Risk and Treatability (START) in acquired brain injury. *Neuropsychological Rehabilitation, 28* (3), 448–465.

Alderman, N., Wood, R.Ll. and Williams, C. (2011). The development of the St Andrew's–Swansea Neurobehavioural Outcome Scale: Validity and reliability of a new measure of neurobehavioural disability and social handicap. *Brain injury, 25* (1), 83–100.

Antaki, C., Barnes, R. and Leudar, I. (2005). Diagnostic formulations in psychotherapy. *Discourse Studies, 7* (6), 627–647.

Beaudoin, M., Potvin, S., Dellazizzo, L., Luigi, M., Giguere, C.E. and Dumais, A. (2019). Trajectories of dynamic risk factors as predictors of violence and criminality in patients discharged from mental health services: A longitudinal study using growth mixture modelling. *Frontiers in Psychiatry, 9* (10), 301.

Boer, D.P., Hart, S.D., Kropp, P.R. and Webster, C.D. (1997). *Manual for the Sexual Violence Risk – 20: Professional Guidelines For Assessing Risk of Sexual Violence*. Burnaby, BC: Mental Health, Law, & Policy Institute, Simon Fraser University.

Carroll, L.J., Cassidy, J.D., Cancelliere, C., Côté, P., Hincapié, C.A., Kristman, V.L., Holm, L.W., Borg, J., Nygren-de Boussard, C., and Hartvigsen, J. (2014). Systematic review of the prognosis after mild traumatic brain injury in adults: Cognitive, psychiatric, and mortality outcomes: Results of the International Collaboration on Mild Traumatic Brain Injury Prognosis. *Archives of Physical Medicine and Rehabilitation, 95* (3 Suppl), S152–S173.

Carswell, K., Maughan, B., Davis, H., Davenport, F. and Goddard, N. (2004). The psychosocial needs of young offenders and adolescents from an inner city area. *Journal of Adolescence*, *27* (4), 415–428.

de Vogel, V., Bruggeman, M. and Lancel, M. (2019). Gender-sensitive violence risk assessment: Predictive validity of six tools in female forensic psychiatric patients. *Criminal Justice and Behaviour*, *46* (4), 528–549.

de Vogel, V., de Vries Robbe, M., van Kalmthout, W. and Place, C. (2012). Risk assessment of violence women: Development of the 'Female Additional Manual' (FAM). *Tijdschrift voor Psychiatrie*, *54* (4), 329–338.

Durrand, V.M. and Crimmins, D.B. (1988). Identifying the variables maintaining self-injurious behaviour. *Journal of Autism & Developmental Disorders*, *18* (1), 99–117.

Ennis, B.J. and Litwack, T.R. (1974). Psychiatry and the presumption of expertise: Flipping coins in the courtroom. *California Law Review*, *62* (3), 693–752.

Garcia-Mansilla, A., Rosenfeld, B. and Cruise, K.R. (2011). Violence risk assessment and women: Predictive accuracy of the HCR-20 in a civil psychiatric hospital. *Behavioural Science and the Law*, *29* (5), 623–633.

Gerald, B., Ortiz, J.B., Green, T.R.F., Brown, S.D., Adelson, P.D., Murphy, S.M. and Rowe, R.K. (2022). Traumatic brain injury characteristics predictive of subsequent sleep-wake disturbances in pediatric patients. *Biology (Basel)*, *11* (4), 600.

Hanson, R.K. (1997). *The Development of a Brief Actuarial Risk Scale for Sexual Offense Recidivism. (User Report 97–04)*. Ottawa, ON: Department of the Solicitor General of Canada.

Harris, G.T., Rice, M.E. and Quinsey, V.L. (1993). Violent recidivism of mentally disordered offenders: The development of a statistical prediction instrument. *Criminal Justice and Behaviour*, *20*, 315–335.

Hart, S., Kropp, P.R. and Laws, D.R., with Klaver, J., Logan, C. and Watt, K.A. (2003). *The Risk for Sexual Violence Protocol (RSVP): Structured Professional Guidelines for Assessing Risk of Sexual Violence*. Vancouver, BC: The Institute Against Family Violence.

Hodgins, S., and Riaz, M. (2011). Violence and phases of illness: Differential risk and predictors. *European Psychiatry*, *26*, 518–524.

Hux, K., Bong, V., Skinner, S., Belau, D. and Sanger, D. (1998). Parental report of occurrences and consequences of traumatic brain injury among delinquent and non-delinquent. *Brain Injury*, *12*, 667–681.

Johnstone, L. and Boyle, M., with Cromby, J., Dillon, J., Harper, D., Kinderman, P., Longden, E., Pilgrim, D. and Read, J. (2018). *The Power Threat Meaning Framework: Towards the Identification of Patterns in Emotional Distress, Unusual Experiences and Troubled or Troubling Behaviour, as an Alternative to Functional Psychiatric Diagnosis*. Leicester: British Psychological Society.

Johnstone, L. and Dallos, R. (2014). *Formulation in Psychology and Psychotherapy: Making Sense of People's Problems*. Abingdon: Routledge.

Katzin, S., Andine, P., Hofvander, B., Billstedt, E. and Wallinus, M. (2020). Exploring traumatic brain injury and aggressive antisocial behaviours in young male violent offenders. *Frontiers in Psychiatry*, *11*, 507196. doi: 10.3389/fpsyt.2020.507196

Lindsay, W.R., Hogue, T.E., Taylor, J.L., Steptoe, L., Mooney, P., O'Brien, G. and Smith, A.H.W. (2008). Risk assessment in offenders with intellectual disability: A comparison across three levels of security. *International Journal of Offender Therapy & Comparative Criminology*, *52*, 90–111.

Mallya, S., Sutherland, J., Pongracic, S., Mainland, B. and Ornstein, T.J. (2015). The manifestation of anxiety disorders after traumatic brain injury: A review. *Journal of Neurotrauma, 32* (7), 411–421.

Marriott, R., O'Shea, L., Picchioni, M.M. and Dickens, G.L. (2017). Predictive validity of the Short-Term Assessment of Risk and Treatability (START) for multiple adverse outcomes: The effect of diagnosis. *Psychiatry Research, 256*, 435–443.

Mooney, P. and Alderman, N. (2022). Assessment of behavioural risk in neurological services. *Neurorehabilitation Times, 23*, https://nrtimes.shorthandstories.com/nr-times-issue-24/neuropsychology/index.html

Morgan, A.B. and Lilienfeld, S.O. (2000). A meta-analytic review of the relation between antisocial behavior and neuropsychological measures of executive function. *Clinical Psychology Review, 20*, 113–136.

Nicholls, T., Gagnon, N., Crocker, A., Brink, J., Desmarais, S. and Webster, C. (2007). *START Outcomes Scale (SOS)*. Vancouver, BC: BC Mental Health & Addiction Services.

Norup, A. and Mortensen, E.L. (2015). Prevalence and predictors of personality change after severe brain injury. *Archives of Physical Medicine and Rehabilitation, 96* (1), 56–62.

Prout, H.T. and Strohmer, D.C. (1991). *Emotional Problems Scales*. Psychological Assessment Resources, Inc.

Rao, V., Rosenberg, P., Bertrand, M., Salehinia, S., Spiro, J., Vaishani, S., Rastogi, P., Noll, K., Schretlen, D.J., Brandt, J., Cornwell, E., Makley, M. and Miles, Q.S. (2009). Aggression after traumatic brain injury: Prevalence and correlates. *Journal of Neuropsychiatry and Clinical Neuroscience, 21* (4), 420–429.

Seligman, M. (2011). *Flourish: A Visionary New Understanding of Happiness and Well-Being*. New York: Free Press.

Shepherd, S.M. and Lewis-Fernandez, R. (2016). Forensic risk assessment and cultural diversity: Contemporary challenges and future directions. *Psychology, Public Policy and Law, 22* (4), 427–438.

Siever, L. (2008). Neurobiology of aggression and violence. *American Journal of Psychiatry, 165* (4), 429–442.

Thornton, D. (2010). *Scoring Guide for Risk Matrix 2000.10/SVC*. Unpublished document.

Thornton, D., Mann, R., Webster, S., Blud, L., Travers, R., Friendship, C. and Erikson, M. (2003). Distinguishing and combining risks for sexual and violent recidivism. In R.A. Prentky, E.S. Janus and M.C. Seto (eds.), *Annals of the New York Academy of Sciences, Sexually Coercive Behavior: Understanding and Management*, Vol. 989 (pp. 225–235). New York: New York Academy of Sciences.

Tonkonogy, J.M. (1991). Violence and temporal love lesion: Head CT and MRI data. *Journal of Neuropsychiatry and Clinical Neuroscience, 3* (2), 189–196.

Tully, J. (2017). HCR-20 shows poor field validity in clinical forensic psychiatry settings. *Evidence Based Mental Health, 20*, 95–96.

Vaishnavi, S., Rao, V. and Fann, J.R. (2009). Neuropsychiatric problems after traumatic brain injury: Unravelling the silent epidemic. *Psychosomatics, 50* (3), 198–205.

Ward, T. (2002). Good lives and the rehabilitation of sexual offenders: Promises and problems. *Aggression and Violent Behavior, 7*, 513–528.

Watts, D., Leese, M., Thomas, S., Atakan, Z. and Wykes, T. (2003). The prediction of violence in acute psychiatric units. *International Journal of Forensic Mental Health, 2*, 173–180.

Webb, T.L. and Sheeran, P. (2006). Does changing behavioral intentions engender behavior change? A meta-analysis of the experimental evidence. *Psychological Bulletin*, *132*, 249–268.

Webster, C.D., Eaves, D., Douglas, K.S. and Wintrup, A. (1995). *The HCR-20 Scheme: The Assessment of Dangerousness and Risk*. British Columbia: Simon Fraser University and British Columbia Forensic Services Commission.

Williams, W.H., Chitsabesan, P., Fazel, S., McMillan, T., Hughes, N., Parsonage, M. and Tonks, J. (2018). Traumatic brain injury: A potential cause of violent crime? *Lancet Psychiatry*, *5* (10), 836–844.

Wood, W., Quinn, J.M. and Kashy, D.A. (2002). Habits in everyday life: Thought, emotion, and action. *Journal of Personality and Social Psychology*, *83*, 1281–1297.

5 Determining the cause

Recording behaviour using direct observation methods

Nick Alderman

Introduction

It will be recalled from the description of the process model in Chapter 2 that the goal of assessment is twofold; first, the identification of variables that maintain challenging behaviour, and, second, the creation of a formulation regarding its function. The formulation equates to a hypothesis regarding the cause of behaviour that subsequently underpins the behaviour support plan evolved to manage this. Chapter 2 described an array of methods to inform this stage of the process, where information is collected from a rich diversity of sources, including interviews, clinical records, and the use of rating scales and questionnaires.

These methods constitute so-called 'proxy' measures in as much as the information they provide comprises indirect measures of behaviour, or of variables that behaviour might reasonably be a product of (for example, attitudes about aggression on a questionnaire, response inhibition on a neuropsychological test).

Reliance on indirect measures for the purpose of formulation constitutes an indirect functional behaviour assessment. However, the likelihood of the subsequent formulation in providing a valid explanation for reasons underpinning challenging behaviour (that in turn provides a strong platform from which to design an effective support plan) is greatly strengthened when an observational functional behaviour assessment is also conducted. This necessitates collecting further information through direct observation of behaviours of concern as they occur in the real world. Practicalities and benefits of directly recording behaviour forms the substance of this chapter, along with description of measurement instruments and methods that the author's experience has shown have particular relevance to management of post-ABI challenging behaviour.

What to measure?

Defining behaviour

Before data collection begins, behaviour that is the subject of assessment must be clearly defined. This requires three criteria to be met. First, it must be possible to ensure behaviour is defined in a way that allows for direct observation.

DOI: 10.4324/9781003083290-7

It cannot comprise some hidden, internal or hypothetical state. The definition must constitute a direct representation of observable characteristics of a person's behaviour as exhibited in the real world. Second, the definition must enable behaviour to be measured in a meaningful way. For example: How often does it take place? How long does it last? Finally, the definition must be articulated so there is a high level of agreement between observers as to when it takes place and when it does not (80 per cent or more) (McHugh, 2012).

The last criterion listed is especially important and should be tested thoroughly before assessment begins, otherwise there is risk that different observers will reach different conclusions regarding whether behaviours of concern have been exhibited across different times and contexts. Lack of agreement between observers introduces measurement error into recordings, leading to under- or over-representation of prevalence; furthermore, it clouds the understanding of relationships between behaviour and potential causal factors, negatively impacting on the formulation and effectiveness of the support plan arising from this.

A good example that illustrates how lack of agreement can impact on estimates of challenging behaviour concerns aggression. We all have some inherent notion of what aggressive behaviour is, but there is no compelling argument that assumes this is universal. In fact, the opposite appears true. In outcome studies examining prevalence of aggression as a post-TBI behaviour disorder, incidence levels vary significantly; for example, in their literature review, Tateno, Jage and Robinson (2003) found the percentage of TBI survivors categorised as 'aggressive' varied from as little as 11 per cent to as much as 96 per cent across different samples; in their study, 34 per cent had engaged in 'significant aggressive behaviour within six months', *as defined by the researchers*. A difficulty underpinning this sizeable variability was recognition of the lack of agreement between researchers regarding a standardised definition of aggression (Alderman, 2015). The need for an agreed definition is equally important when an individual person is being rated by multiple observers. Whilst the clinician leading assessment may have a very clear idea of what 'aggression' means to them, it cannot be assumed this others share this. For example, some people may interpret 'aggression' as solely comprising physical assaults on others, while others may employ wider criteria and record verbal insults, shouting and non-verbal aspects, such as staring, fist-clenching and invasion of personal space.

Regarding clinical management, data integrity should be sufficient to reliably track response to rehabilitation over time using SCED methodology (see Chapter 2). The target behaviour comprises the dependent variable, recordings of which are used for multiple purposes, including determining the impact of treatment interventions through quantitative comparison of no-treatment, or baseline, periods with times when interventions are in operation. Defining behaviours to record using imprecise concepts, such as 'violence', 'irritability' and 'agitation', are inadequate. It is also important to distinguish between different types of aggression to achieve consistent reporting. Without this, measurement error arising from lack of agreement between observers will undermine the ability to meaningfully determine outcomes of behaviour support plans.

When thinking about minimising measurement error, the three key psychometric properties of validity, reliability and responsiveness also equate to key criteria required in defining behaviour recorded through direct observation. A definition must be:

a valid – that is, observable – in providing an *accurate representation* of the behaviour of interest;
b reliable – that is, achieve agreement between observers – multiple observers *recognise and agree* when behaviour has been exhibited; and
c possess responsiveness – that is, be measurable – it can be applied to consistently *measure change over time and context* in this behaviour.

Successful utilisation of these key scientific properties escalates a description to an *operational definition of behaviour* because it can be clearly observed, measured regardless of time or context, and observers are in agreement about when it is and when it is not exhibited.

Other pre-assessment considerations

Other considerations also need to be taken into account when planning assessment. First, context. Observations should be collected within the context where behaviour naturally occurs. It may be behaviours are more likely to take place at certain times of the day, or within certain activities. Steps to determine if behaviours have situational specificity should form part of the initial assessment. This will be readily identifiable when there is a continuous system of measurement in place, such as the partial interval recording method described later. Assessment should include as many contexts as possible that the person is routinely exposed to, to ensure records made are representative. If behaviour is found to have high situational specificity (for example, if it is only observed in particular therapy sessions), then resources can be allocated to collect more detailed records at these times.

Sometimes behaviours occur so infrequently that maintaining continuous observation is redundant. A solution is to determine conditions that elicit behaviour by experimentally manipulating various antecedents and consequences using the framework provided by experimental functional analysis (see Chapter 2). This solution should also be applied when there are difficulties in observing behaviour under natural conditions (for example, because of risk or level of intrusiveness).

A second pre-assessment point to consider is *who* should collect behaviour data? When continuous observation is employed, there are advantages in expecting all members of the clinical team to make recordings whenever required. There will, however, be challenges in fulfilling this expectation, and having a pool of designated observers available may provide a solution.

A third point to contemplate is that all observers must be trained to ensure the validity of recordings. Training ensures there is shared understanding of the operational definition of behaviour and the methods used to collect information. The operational definition will articulate behaviour using objective, observable criteria; confirmation should be sought that everybody is able to correctly identify behaviour. First, a written description of the operational definition must be clearly provided in the behaviour support plan. Second, the extent of agreement between observers should be ascertained (for example, by asking people individually what the behaviour comprises and then comparing responses). A lack of agreement indicates the operational definition of behaviour requires rewriting and testing until observers successfully identify this (at least 80 per cent agreement between raters) (see McHugh, 2012). Discussion, role play and video recordings of actual incidents can facilitate this. Observers must also be trained in the use of measurement instruments and methods (these will be discussed later).

A final pre-assessment consideration concerns 'drift', a tendency for observers to deviate from the agreed operational definition of behaviour over time that can be attributed to fatigue, forgetting, loss of motivation and subtle changes in the behaviour itself (Girard and Cohn, 2016). This is mediated through repeated training and discussion. Accuracy may improve when observers are conscious of being monitored. 'Reactivity' occurs when individuals change behaviour because they are aware they are being observed. Whilst this may improve recordings, the person being observed should not be aware of being monitored as this will change their behaviour too. Observers need to be discreet regarding proximity and actions. This may be less of an issue in contexts where a lot of overt records are made, such as in a hospital setting, but generally consideration needs to be given regarding the balance between discretion and making accurate records.

How to measure?

Having decided what to measure, decisions regarding how and when data can be collected need to be made. Paper records are most likely to be used. They can be mounted on clipboards carried by an observer or available in some accessible central location when this is a team task.

Continuous recording

One option is to continually observe and maintain a written record of behaviour. Making an audio record through the observer describing what they see and hear using a digital voice recorder may be an option, although time will need to be spent transcribing outputs from this. It may also be less discreet. Written and audio records generate a rich, minute-by-minute detailed log of a person's activities. These can be helpful in highlighting behaviours that will require subsequent detailed specific monitoring using other means of recording.

Making a very detailed record of behaviour using continuous observation has some potential drawbacks that need careful consideration beforehand. First, it is staff intensive, requiring an observer to be delegated to this task, and this task alone, for a fixed period. In busy clinical teams with a high workload this may not be possible; however, it might be manageable if the person being monitored is on continuous observation to maintain their safety and the safety of others and are accompanied by at least one member of staff who can take on this additional function. Second, further resources must be made available to review written records and extract key information. This process usually necessitates two or more clinicians independently studying records to minimise possible bias in selection of behaviours of concern that might be subject to more detailed assessment. Third, caution and skill are required by observers making ongoing records about a person's behaviour, as being seen to follow, observe and make records may induce reactivity through 'observer effect', as described earlier. Observer behaviours may arouse suspicion and even paranoia, which must be avoided. A fourth point to consider is observer fatigue arising from continuously observing and recording a person's behaviour. The regular, frequent substitution of observers, perhaps on an hourly basis, will help minimise this.

Despite these potential difficulties, continuous recording is most practical and useful when assessing people who exhibit very little overt behaviour, perhaps because of an arousal or drive disorder, or because of difficulties with initiation. In these cases, when people do engage in the behaviour or activity of concern, it can be overlooked; so having a designated system of observers in place for a fixed period of assessment will help ensure the smallest actions are recorded.

Time-sampling

A method that reduces the impact of many of these issues is time-sampling. This refers to a variety of methods employed to record behaviour at specific moments. Although most of these have relevance to capturing information about behaviour in clinical work with people with ABI, one or two have special practical relevance.

In the experience of the author, the most frequent use of time-sampling is where the person is closely observed for one or more defined periods each day. This is undertaken to the point where sufficient periods of observation are accumulated to be representative of the person's behaviour. Observations are planned in advance, with a typical duration of 30 minutes or 1 hour. If the intent is to draw conclusions about behaviour occurring regardless of time or context, then the advance planning needs to randomise observation periods that are representative of all the activities undertaken (for example, attending meals, rehabilitation sessions, leisure time). An eight-hour time-sample might be conducted over the course of a few days, with two or more observation periods each day, conducted at quasi-random times (so there is no overlap).

As well as being more practical and requiring less resource than continuous measurement, time-sampling is well suited to determine success of treatment interventions. For example, Alderman and Ward (1991) described reduction of verbal perseveration that prevented the rehabilitation of AB, a 36-year-old female who had sustained an ABI through contracting the herpes simplex encephalitis virus. Intervention was undertaken in 50 daily one-hour sessions. Whilst SCED methodology clearly demonstrated improvement within sessions, these records could not guarantee generalisation outside the sessions, or that gains would be maintained. Time-sampling answered these questions. In the week before intervention, a baseline of the frequency of repetitive speech (defined as immediate repetition of a word, phrase or sentence) was undertaken where AB was observed for two half-hour periods per day over five consecutive days. Sampling was constructed so that half the observations were made during therapy sessions, the rest at other times. This was repeated for the week immediately following the withdrawal of the intervention, and again three months later. Recordings confirmed the likelihood that gains made in sessions had generalised and persisted; a total of 985 episodes of verbal perseveration were recorded during the five-hour period pre-intervention, 253 in the first week post-intervention, and 149 three months later. In addition to evidence of maintenance, breaking recordings down further suggested benefits had generalised across contexts too.

Frequency vs severity vs duration recording

Behaviour recordings made in neurorehabilitation often reflect frequency, a count of how many times a behaviour is observed over a specific time. Using a clear operational definition of the behaviour, this can provide a robust, valid, reliable measure. However, sometimes a frequency count alone fails to convey important characteristics of behaviour. For example, incidence of physical aggression against other people may not change over time, leading to a conclusion that a behaviour support plan had not been ineffective. However, whilst frequency remains unaffected, severity may have reduced. A more robust set of measurements will be obtained by collecting two data sets, counting how often aggression took place and quantifying severity of behaviour, perhaps using a 5-point scale. Alternatively, employing separate operational definitions that reflect various levels of severity also provides a reliable means of discriminating change in complex behaviours; this is best achieved using an observational recording measure, which will be discussed later in this chapter.

Another important characteristic of behaviour that will not be captured adequately by counting how often it occurs, is duration – how long it lasts for. Many challenging behaviours constitute short-lived, distinct episodes, but others may be prolonged, or less easy to differentiate regarding when they start and end. Examples of prolonged behaviours that may be more challenging than suggested by frequency counts alone include shouting, wailing, head banging, laying on the floor, sleeping, disengagement from therapy activities, staring and pacing. A frequency count of any of these might be low, but this would not adequately capture the true impact a behaviour has, as each 'count' may last minutes or hours. When this is the case, having an observation metric that reflects duration is highly desirable.

Measure using what?

Some specific ways of recording behaviour that the author has found to be especially relevant in working with people with post-ABI challenging behaviour will now be described, along with advice regarding associated benefits and drawbacks.

Partial interval recording

This method can be used to obtain behaviour recordings throughout the day. Typically, a grid is drawn on A4 paper, with columns representing days of the week, further subdivided each day into defined time periods, for example 15-minute blocks. Behaviours to be recorded can be assigned a shorthand code (for example, NC meaning 'non-cooperation'). When any of these behaviours are observed, the code can be recorded within the appropriate box on the form. See Figure 5.1 for an example of this.

15 Minute Behaviour Recording Sheet

Please enter the code(s) for the following behaviours for any 15-minute period in which they have been observed at least once: VA – Verbal Aggression; PA – Physical Aggression; NC – Non-compliance with prompts. Please tick the box for any 15-minute period in which none of these behaviours are observed.

Name __Nick Alderman__   w/c __26/7__

	MON		TUES		WED		THURS		FRI		SAT		SUN	
08.15 – 08.30	✓	✓ VA PA	VA	VA	VA	✓	VA NC	✓	PA	PA	VA	✓	✓	VA
08.45 – 09.00	✓	VA	VA	PA	✓	✓	✓	NC	PA NC	✓	✓	✓	VA	✓
09.15 – 09.30	✓	✓	VA PA	✓	✓	VA	✓	✓	✓	VA	✓	✓	✓	✓
09.45 – 10.00	PA NC	✓	✓	NC	VA	VA	VA	✓	✓	✓	✓	✓	✓	✓
10.15 – 10.30	✓	✓	NC	✓	✓	VA	✓	✓	✓	✓	✓	✓	✓	✓
10.45 – 11.00	✓	PA	✓	NC	NC	✓	✓	NC	✓	✓	✓	VA	✓	✓
11.15 – 11.30	✓	PA	✓	✓	✓	VA	✓	NC	✓	✓	✓	✓	✓	VA
11:45 – 12.00	✓	✓	✓	VA	✓	✓	✓	✓	✓	PA	✓	✓	VA	✓

Figure 5.1 Example of a partial interval recording form designed to capture behaviour data throughout the day. Only the part of the form reflecting the early part of the day is shown for illustrative purposes. Indices extracted from recordings for the period shown include 21 verbal aggression, 11 physical aggression and 10 non-cooperation. Note these figures do not reflect discrete frequencies but, instead, 15-minute periods in which behaviours recorded were observed at least once. No target behaviours were observed in 75 of the 112 15-minute periods observed, which provides a further index of 66.9 per cent appropriate behaviour.

Advantages are that this method provides a continuous record, highlighting behaviours of concern, and it also tracks the occurrence of these over time. Potential relationships between behaviour and time of day may become apparent. It is a simple method and therefore more likely to be reliable. A range of useful indices can be generated. For example: a total weekly count of each behaviour; and a proxy measure of appropriate behaviour expressed as a percentage of 15-minute (or equivalent) periods in which no observations were recorded, over the total number of time-intervals available (number observation periods no behaviour recorded/total number observation periods <x> 100). Regular review of these indices helps raise awareness of behaviours requiring detailed assessment as well as tracking the response to rehabilitation. A limitation of the approach is a lack of sensitivity – the records only confirm that behaviours of interest were exhibited during a 15-minute period (or whatever time is decided), but they cannot testify to the exact frequency, and they say nothing regarding severity and duration. A further potential drawback is that this approach is usually reliant on any member of the clinical team making a recording, as and when the designated behaviours occur; compliance will need to be monitored to maintain accurate recordings.

Despite these shortfalls, partial interval recording provides a reasonable and simple means of compiling a continuous record of behaviour that may be sufficient to highlight need and track change over time.

Tally chart

A simple method to record frequency counts is the tally chart. This can take the form of a printed sheet broken down into days, times and activities, as needed. When a certain behaviour is observed, a tick is made in the appropriate space. Tally charts enable continuous recording of the frequency of behaviour from which totals are extracted in whatever way is meaningful and useful indices constructed. For example, collecting observations every hour throughout the day for seven days enables total frequency for the week and calculation of the average frequency per day and hour. Tally charts can also be employed in time-sampling. When a dedicated observer is used, increased discretion can be facilitated by dispensing with the clipboard, printed sheet and pen and using a tally counter that fits snugly in the hand (see 'Applications of technology' section later). At the end of the observation session, the number of counts made can then be recorded separately. An example of a tally chart is shown in Figure 5.2.

A tally chart is especially useful in recording high frequency, discrete behaviours. A potential shortfall is that, because behaviours may be frequent, a dedicated observer is sometimes required.

Measurement of frequency and duration

Methods that provide concurrent indices regarding frequency and duration of behaviour are necessarily more complex, and for this reason inevitably require a dedicated observer using time-sampling.

Name: Nick Alderman	Behaviour to Record: Non-cooperation	
Date	Tally	Total
26.07.21	✓✓✓✓	4
27.07.21	✓✓✓✓✓✓✓✓ ✓✓✓✓	12
28.07.21	✓✓	2
29.07.21	✓	1
30.07.21		0

Figure 5.2 Example of a tally chart in which a simple record of the daily frequency of non-cooperation has been obtained.

Partial interval recording was described earlier but there are variants that can be usefully employed. First, *whole interval recording*. The period of observation is subdivided into smaller intervals of equal length, for example 30 seconds. This is translated onto a sheet for recording purposes, 30 sec, 1 min, 1 min 30 secs, etc. At the start of observation, the observer initiates a stopwatch and closely monitors this. If the target behaviour has been evident throughout the whole of the current interval a tick mark is placed alongside that to indicate this, a cross if not (for example, if behaviour occurred continuously for the period 1 min to 1 min 30 secs, then a tick is placed against 1 min 30 secs on the form; if it had not been observed at all, a cross would be recorded instead). Afterwards, the percentage of intervals in which behaviour was observed is determined. The resulting metric provides a useful means of capturing both frequency and duration, but it also requires extreme vigilance on the part of the observer. A further variant of interval recording is *momentary time-sampling*. Here, the observer records behaviour has taken place when this is observed at the exact time of each interval (for example, the observer only records a tick against 1 min 30 secs if the behaviour was noted to be evident *at this exact time*). This is less likely to tire an observer, but it compromises increased reliability with a less sensitive measure.

The final method provides the best quality information, combining benefits of 'how many and for how long?'. However, practice is required to become proficient as it involves manual dexterity and good coordination. In *frequency/ duration recording*, the observer adds a stopwatch to their paper-and-pen record. First, the time observation begins is noted and the stopwatch activated. Whenever a behaviour of interest is observed, the time elapsed from the stopwatch is noted under a 'start' column; similarly, when it is no longer evident, that time is recorded on the same line under a 'finish' column. Afterwards, total frequency is evident from the number of 'start/finish' pairs; and an average 'how long' (duration) index can be calculated by dividing the total time spent engaged in the behaviour by frequency. Similarly, the total time can be divided by the length of the observation period and the result multiplied by 100 to obtain the percentage of the session engaged in the target behaviour.

FREQUENCY/DURATION RECORDING

Name: __Nick Alderman__

Behaviour to record: __Shouting – see care plan for operational definition__

Session start:__10:00____ Session finished:__10:20____

Start	Stop	Duration
1'40"	2'18"	38"
3'15"	4'32"	77"
5'22"	8'13"	171"
10'11"	15'18"	307"
16'00"	19'02"	182"
	Total Duration	775"
	Session Duration	1200"

Figure 5.3 Example of a frequency/duration recording form used to capture information about shouting in rehabilitation sessions. Several useful indices can be generated from these data to help evaluate effectiveness of subsequent interventions to reduce shouting (see text).

An example of frequency/duration recording is shown in Figure 5.3. The relevant metrics are calculated from the recordings made, including the average duration of the target behaviour (775 secs/5 = 155 secs, or 2 mins 35 secs) and the percentage of the total time spent engaged in shouting ([775 secs/1200 secs] <x> 100 = 64.6 per cent).

Given the complex multitasking required for this form of observation, it only makes sense to use it when frequency is moderate or less, otherwise reliability is undermined by the amount of data logged. A very practised, deft observer might go about this differently, ditching the clipboard and paper-and-pen in favour of a tally counter in one hand and stopwatch in the other. When behaviour occurs, the observer can record this on the counter while pressing the 'start' function on the stopwatch and the 'stop' function when the behaviour ends. Afterwards, total frequency is evident from the tally counter, and total time engaged in behaviour from the stopwatch. This information is used to calculate the same indices as the paper-and-pen/stopwatch method.

ABC charts

A limitation inherent in the recording methods described so far is that, except for time of day, no information is captured that can meaningfully contribute to a functional assessment regarding determinants of behaviour.

One response to this is use of the 'ABC chart', which provides a method of recording behaviour directly informed by the operant learning framework. This extends information captured to include environmental variables that may reinforce or otherwise influence its occurrence. Principal features and their relevance to functional assessment are plain when the acronym is expanded: 'A' represents 'Antecedent', the last event observed immediately prior to the behaviour of interest; 'B' equates to describing the 'Behaviour' itself; and 'C' represents its 'Consequences', the last event observed before the behaviour stopped. Additional information typically included on the chart includes the date and time behaviour was observed. An example of a completed ABC chart is shown in Figure 5.4.

ABC charts are flexible and can be used in a variety of applications. For example, when a patient is first admitted, a chart can be employed for members of the clinical team to record behaviours of note that can then be followed up for further discussion. Behaviours captured using the partial interval recording method described can also be investigated further using ABC charts. They can also be modified to facilitate collection of additional information relevant to an individual, and can be employed by an observer conducting a functional assessment in a specific context – for example, aggression exhibited in a physiotherapy session.

Whilst ABC charts are undoubtedly helpful in highlighting behaviours for further investigation, they should not be relied on as the only means of behaviour recording. First, there is no guarantee that 'behaviours of note' will necessarily be consistently logged by members of a busy clinical team, who may hold

ABC Chart

Please use this chart to make records about any challenging behaviour.

Name ___Nick Alderman_____   w/c ___26/7___

Time & Date	ANTECEDENT *What happened immediately before the behaviour?*	BEHAVIOUR *What behaviour occurred?*	CONSEQUENCE *What happened immediately after the behaviour?*
27/7/21 2:15pm	Reminded NA it would soon be time to attend physio session.	NA shouted at me to go away and leave him alone.	I downplayed NA's behaviour and did not respond directly to it.
2:17pm	Prompted NA that he should make his way down to physio.	NA told me to "f_off" and raised his fist at me.	I left the room and informed the nurse-in-charge.

Figure 5.4 An example of an ABC chart.

disparate views on what should be recorded as 'challenging' behaviour. Second, the level of detail of information varies between observers. Third, instead of providing an objective record of what was observed, observer bias can degrade the quality of recordings. In short, ABC chart information has unknown reliability and validity.

This can be improved by pre-populating the 'Behaviour' column with a robust operational definition to increase the likelihood that observations are limited to behaviours of interest. However, at some point, other, more robust, measures should be introduced to obtain more dependable measures and other procedures employed to undertake functional assessment.

Observational recording measures

Observational recording measures (ORM) are characterised by strengths that render them powerful tools for collection of data regarding behaviour and functional assessment (see Girard and Cohn, 2016). Particularly important is the ability to minimise observer measurement error by focusing attention on specific behaviours and variables of interest, choosing responses from standardised lists in which items are operationally defined, and recording behaviour through assignment to discrete categories, or rating them on continuous dimensions. ORMs transform observations of behaviour into quantitative judgements; consequently, good measures have known psychometric properties and, therefore, confidence that data are valid and reliable. Furthermore, they are derived from and inform specific theories of behaviour, including learning theory. For our purpose, ORMs that have special relevance are those that, like ABC charts, are underpinned by an operant learning framework. However, unlike ABC charts, observers make quantitative judgements about behaviours of interest which reliably capture the unfolding of behaviour over time and, through this, gain an understanding of its function.

Examples of two ORMs developed specifically for ABI are the 'Overt Aggression Scale – Modified for Neurorehabilitation' (OAS-MNR) (Alderman, Knight and Morgan, 1997) and the 'St Andrew's Sexual Behaviour Assessment' (SASBA) (Knight et al., 2008). Both instruments were developed as a response to the lack of standardised definitions and measures regarding aggression and inappropriate sexual behaviour (ISB). The OAS-MNR was developed from the Overt Aggression Scale (Yudofsky et al., 1986), a well-known measure of aggressive behaviour observed in the psychiatric context; and in turn, the SASBA was developed as an extension of the OAS-MNR for the measurement of ISB.

Both measures offer an identical framework for translating what an observer sees and hears into a set of standardised written descriptors, organised into four categories of behaviour, each of which are further organised into four levels of severity, from 'mild' to 'very severe' equating to a numerical scale from 1 to 4. Quantifiable metrics are generated regarding type of behaviour, frequency and severity. Information to help understand function is also collected regarding 3 potential setting events, 15 immediate antecedents and 14 interventions, enabling the production of further indices. A series of codes for setting events, antecedents, type of aggression and severity, and interventions (numbers and letters) are defined in a reference sheet used to document observations on a recording sheet, providing a shorthand means of reliably capturing complex behaviour sequences. As only behaviour descriptions differ between OAS-MNR and SASBA, both can be employed using the same recording form, providing a comprehensive means of capturing sequences of action as they unfold. The reference and recording forms are available on request from the author.

An example of behaviour recordings made using OAS-MNR is shown in Figure 5.5. The first two columns of the recording sheet enable date and time of aggression to be noted, enabling the chronological unfolding of behaviour to be understood. Next, initials of the observer are written, in case further information is required. The next four columns are concerned with antecedent data. If aggression takes place in the context of any of three 'setting events' – variables that do not directly trigger behaviour but may increase likelihood it occurs – then a tick is placed in the relevant column(s) to confirm this. The fourth column is always completed as it is here the event directly observed to precede behaviour is noted. Next, codes for type and severity of aggression are recorded, followed by a column to note the intervention observed that ended the aggressive behaviour. Space is provided in the final column to place a tick for every subsequent episode of aggression, which has identical codes, that takes place very shortly afterwards, eliminating the need to replicate these in full.

So, in the first line of the reference sheet, aggression was observed on 11 June at 10:25 am; this took place in a 'structured activity', as confirmed by a tick in the relevant column (neither of the other two setting events applied), and the immediate antecedent was '11' – the person was 'Given a direct verbal prompt to comply with an instruction'. Type of aggression was VA (Verbal Aggression of 'mild'

OVERT AGGRESSION SCALE – MODIFIED FOR NEUROREHABILITATION (OAS-MNR)
Alderman, Knight & Morgan, 1997

Name: Nick Alderman

			Antecedents						
			Contributing Factors -tick if applies			Observed Directly Beforehand (1-25)	Aggression (type, rating)	Intervention (A-N)	Multiple Recordings*
Date	Time	Observer Initials	Structured Activity	Noisy Environment	Epilepsy prev 24 hrs				
11/06	10:25	CK	✓			11	VA1	A	✓✓✓
11/06	10:30	CK	✓			22	PP2	L	

Figure 5.5 Examples of consecutive behaviour recordings made using the OAS-MNR. The use of codes enables shorthand recording of unfolding complex behaviour sequences, making a major contribution to understanding what functions behaviour serves, as well as providing quantitative information used to help determine effectiveness of treatment.

severity; 1 is compatible with 'Makes loud noise, shouts angrily, is not person directed, for example *bloody hell*'). The intervention that ended this behaviour was A (Behaviour ignored or 'played down' completely). The final column contains four ticks, confirming the same behaviour sequence was observed in rapid succession, indicating five episodes of mild verbal aggression had taken place over a short period. The second line of the form shows some escalation in behaviour from verbal to physical aggression against people (PP) five minutes later. Severity was 'moderate' (2) corresponding to 'Strikes, kicks, pushes, pulls hair, without significant injury'. This occurred in structured activity, triggered by the person's 'Purposeful behaviour (being) ignored or "played down" by the person to whom it was directed'. The intervention that ended this behaviour was use of an individually designed programme (L, Special programme).

The contribution of ORMs to understanding the function of behaviour is apparent in just these two lines of recordings: the person was being prompted to complete a task in a rehabilitation session; mild verbal aggression did not result in withdrawal of prompts and the behaviour escalated to the therapist being physically assaulted. Interpretation of these data suggest a formulation in which verbal aggression had previously been negatively reinforced as it led to avoidance or escape from rehabilitation sessions; and that aggressive behaviour escalated as the reinforcer associated with verbal aggression was withheld as prompting continued, conforming to the expectation of the operant phenomena of extinction, when a reinforcer (withdrawal of demands) is withheld.

ORMs have many advantages. They can be employed in time-sampling observations, or in situations where continuous recording is required – perhaps following a period of partial interval observation in which frequent aggression has been noted and more detailed information is recorded. Operational definitions of behaviour equip clinicians with a standardised vocabulary that helps shared objectivity and reduced observer bias. They also make a direct, seamless contribution to understanding drivers of behaviour, being employed in both observational functional behaviour assessment and experimental functional analysis. Possible drawbacks of using ORMs is the commitment to training all members of the clinical team in how to use them. Time and resources also need to be committed to collate and analyse recordings. ORMs are also not available for all types of challenging behaviour associated with ABI outcomes.

ORMs have additional benefits above individual clinical work; for example, both the OAS-MNR and SASBA have made meaningful contributions to service evaluation, clinical audit, benchmarking with other services, research and marketing (for example, see Alderman and Knight, 2017).

Applications of technology

Tally counters

Various technology applications assist and enhance the direct recording of behaviour. The most primitive is the use of tally counters, of which there are two types, mechanical and digital. These are typically employed in sports and industrial applications but are also indispensable in behaviour recording. The mechanical variant typically consists of a metal chassis mounting an external switch and 4-digit counter; the counter advances when the switch is pressed. Digital versions can be very small and offer various programmable functions. Both types are compact and easily concealed within a closed hand. Whereas mechanical devices invariably make an audible 'click' when used, their digital counterparts can be set either to emit an audible confirmation or to offer a silent mode. In most applications, the ability to make a silent recording will be preferable, but there are some instances when an audible alert is desirable – for example, in interventions designed to increase awareness.

Video recording

A second 'low-tech' application is video recording. Whilst previously the domain of expensive equipment, with the advent of high-quality video recording on smartphones this is now an affordable option. However, there may be legal and other constraints on who and what can be recorded, and on the usage and storage of material. There are considerable advantages. For example, contexts in which challenging behaviour is highly likely to occur can be filmed; episodes of behaviour can be viewed in detail many times to glean maximum information. Having two or more devices filming simultaneously from different locations enables incidents to be viewed from different angles and distances, providing more sources of information. The use of video in training observers to consistently recognise behaviour was mentioned earlier. This can be extended in several ways. For example, multiple observers can independently view the same video clips and record behaviour; these can be compared to determine the degree of agreement (the extent to which recordings are identical) across observers using a number of indices, from a simple percentage agreement or correlation coefficient, to more sophisticated statistical methods enabling the comparison of recordings made by three or more observers, such as Fleiss's Kappa (Fleiss, 1971) and the intraclass correlation coefficient (see Howell, 1997, pp. 490–493).

Video recordings can also be employed to help quantify observers' perceptions about aspects of behaviour that are not directly observable, but that nevertheless contribute towards the formulation, or they can be used as further measures to help determine treatment outcomes. For example, Alderman, Shepherd and Youngson (1992) used six independent observers to view two video recordings of participation in sessions made before and after a behaviour support plan was implemented; the order in which the recordings were presented was randomised to minimise bias. Observers used a 10-point scale to rate seven items reflecting the patients behavioural and affective state (for example, avoidance of the task, distress and anxiety experienced, cooperation with the task). Comparison of mean ratings indicated improvement across six of the seven items, providing further evidence of the benefits of the support plan in addition to the reduction in directly observable challenging behaviour.

Audio recording

Technology can also assist in identifying when behaviours occur by providing external means of validation, triggered when a threshold is met. An example of this is speech volume. Burgess and Alderman (1990) described the case of a 60-year-old TBI survivor who presented with a range of neurocognitive impairments, including poor memory, marked perseveration and reduced inhibitory control. A behaviour that interfered with his rehabilitation was the volume of his normal speaking voice, which was so loud that he became unmanageable in a group setting. Relying solely on a written definition of what constituted an inappropriate volume for normal conversation proved insufficient. In addition, the patient had difficulty monitoring this aspect of his behaviour, so a further method of providing a reliable means of indicating this was occurring was required. An audio recorder and microphone were placed on the desk at a fixed distance from the patient. An integral component within the audio recorder was a large VU meter; this responded to the volume of sound detected by the microphone and resulted in the needle moving across its face; the background colour of the meter went from green (no sound) to red (maximum volume) and was normally calibrated to maximise the quality of the audio recording by reducing background noise and 'clipping' resulting from excess volume. For the purpose of intervention, no audio recording was made, but the sensitivity of the VU meter was calibrated such that the needle would go beyond a fixed point, marked with a piece of coloured sticking tape. During sessions, in which the patient read single words, short phrases and sentences, a therapist monitored the meter and was able to consistently make recordings that discriminated the number of verbal utterances spoken within the acceptable volume range and those that exceeded this threshold. Part of the intervention that followed entailed the patient using the VU meter to monitor the volume of his voice; this was sufficiently successful to explore the use of a microphone headset the patient could wear throughout the day to help him monitor speech volume and generalise the positive results from the sessional work throughout the day.

Digital recording

Digital recording platforms have many advantages. Digital tablets are increasingly used in healthcare settings and are perceived as part of the normal paraphernalia, minimising observer reactivity. Digital versions of behaviour records lend themselves well to touch-screen applications, resulting in faster, more efficient completion. Difficulties arising from poor handwriting are eliminated; and missing items are less likely as applications often require the full information set to be entered before information can be submitted. Problems with storing paper copies are resolved. Tablet applications are ideally linked into a network and data automatically backed up; some applications directly interface with a database or statistical software, eliminating the laborious task of manually transferring recordings from paper copies onto a computer. This ensures the latest information is always accessible and can be shared effectively within the clinical team. At least one provider has moved from pen-and-paper to digital application of the OAS-MNR, using tablets, with data being immediately available in this way (I. Stewart, personal communication, 12 May 2020).

Rahman and colleagues (Rahman, Oliver and Alderman, 2010; Rahman, Alderman and Oliver, 2013) utilised handheld personal computers running observational software that enabled convenient recording of individualised behaviours and environmental events. These provided a high degree of analytical detail, sufficient to undertake comprehensive structured descriptive assessments with benefits over and above traditional means of recording behaviour. For example, in their investigation of challenging behaviour in four people who had sustained ABI, a reliable measure of functional relationships was obtained with a mean assessment duration of just 2.25 hours per person.

There are some potential pitfalls to using digital technology. Start-up costs may prove prohibitive. Tablets are not immune to damage so require additional protection to ensure they are robust enough. They may go missing and there is a risk that expensive technology may be lost. Battery life also needs consideration: safeguards need to be in place to ensure regular charging while ensuring sufficient devices are available for use 24/7. Finally, data may also be vulnerable to loss through equipment failure, so a backup system is required.

Integrating direct observation methods into the process model

There is a useful spread of direct observation methods and measures available to the practitioner that informs functional behaviour assessment and formulation regarding the reasons underpinning challenging behaviour. It would make no sense to utilise all of these; instead, careful selection of those methods that best match the clinical model and organisation of a service is required.

Drawing on the experience of the author, the following description of how direct observation methods best compliment the process model in working with post-ABI challenging behaviour are briefly described.

1 Use the partial interval recording method to collect continuous data at the start of assessment; supplement with ABC charts to enable others to record potential behaviours of interest. Conder use of continuous recording in the case of individuals who emit little obvious behaviour.
2 Review these data and decide what behaviours, if any, require further assessment. For those that do, produce operational definitions of behaviour and test these to ensure all involved share an identical understanding of what these are. These enable generation of quantitative metrics relevant to that behaviour, that is, frequency, severity, duration. Consider other pre-assessment considerations and decide how observations are collected, including the use of technology, where available. If assessment suggests situational specificity, direct observation methods will be capable of distinguishing times,

settings and contexts when behaviour peaks. If this is not evident, time-sampling should be employed across the range of contexts behaviour occurs.
3 Measurement instruments, and the methodologies used to deploy them, should carry on being used in the same way throughout the time the behaviour support plan is in operation. This will enable target behaviours to be consistently tracked using direct observation, and will allow a valid comparison of different stages of a plan to be determined.
4 The use of ORMs is particularly recommended as they will generate appropriate metrics and a range of other useful information that can inform both observational functional assessment and experimental functional analysis.

Summary and practical implications

Direct observation of challenging behaviour provides essential information that informs assessment and enables reliable responses to support plans to be determined. Operational definitions of behaviour ensure validity through agreement within clinical teams regarding what constitutes challenging behaviour through the enablement of individual bespoke parameters. Methods are available that enable quantifiable indices to be generated regarding frequency, severity and duration, as appropriate. Metrics concerning frequency, severity and duration of challenging behaviours are used in the assessment stage to compile a baseline. Ongoing capture of the same information during intervention enables the success of the methods used to be determined; and, following this, further collection of the same indices will indicate to what extent treatment effects have sustained and generalised to other contexts.

The use of ORMs is particularly recommended as they will generate appropriate metrics and a range of other useful information that can inform both observational functional assessment and experimental functional analysis. Their psychometric properties offer additional safeguards. Further confidence comes from utilising instruments conceptualised for use with ABI populations. Looking ahead, provision of these instruments on a digital platform promises additional advantages regarding efficiency and reliability, especially with regard to data integrity, security and analyses. Such developments are awaited with eager anticipation.

References

Alderman, N. (2015). Acquired brain injury, trauma and aggression. In G. Dickens, M. Picchioni and P. Sugarman (eds), *Handbook of Specialist Secure Patient Mental Healthcare*. London: The Royal College of Psychiatrists.
Alderman, N., Knight, C. and Morgan, C. (1997). Use of a modified version of the Overt Aggression Scale in the measurement and assessment of aggressive behaviours following brain injury. *Brain Injury*, *11*, 503–523.
Alderman, N. and Knight, C. (2017). Keeping the 'scientist-practitioner' model alive and kicking through service-based evaluation and research: Examples from neurobehavioural rehabilitation. *The Neuropsychologist*, *3* (April), 25–32.

Alderman, N., Shepherd, J. and Youngson, H.A. (1992). Increasing standing tolerance and posture quality following severe brain injury using a behaviour modification approach. *Physiotherapy, 78*, 335–343.

Alderman, N. and Ward, A. (1991). Behavioural treatment of the dysexecutive syndrome: Reduction of repetitive speech using response cost and cognitive overlearning. *Neuropsychological Rehabilitation, 1*, 65–80.

Burgess, P.W. and Alderman, N. (1990). Rehabilitation of dyscontrol syndromes following frontal lobe damage: A cognitive neuropsychological approach. In R.Ll. Wood and I. Fussey (ed.), *Cognitive Rehabilitation in Perspective*. Basingstoke: Taylor & Francis.

Fleiss, J. L. (1971). Measuring nominal scale agreement among many raters. *Psychological Bulletin, 76*, 378–382.

Girard, J.M. and Cohn, J.F. (2016). A primer on observational measurement. *Assessment, 23*, 404–413.

Howell, D.C. (1997). *Statistical Methods for Psychology* (4th edn). Belmont, CA: Duxbury Press.

Knight, C., Alderman, N., Johnson, C., Green, S., Birkett-Swan, L. and Yorston, G. (2008). The St Andrew's Sexual Behaviour Assessment (SASBA): Development of a standardised recording instrument for the measurement and assessment of challenging sexual behaviour in people with progressive and acquired neurological impairment. *Neuropsychological Rehabilitation, 18*, 129–159.

McHugh, M. (2012). Interrater reliability: The Kappa statistic. *Biochemia Medica, 22*, 276–282.

Rahman, B., Alderman, N. and Oliver, C. (2013). The application of a structured descriptive assessment methodology with traumatic brain injury survivors to identify the function of challenging behaviour. *Neuropsychological Rehabilitation: An International Journal, 23*, 501–527. DOI:10.1080/09602011.2013.787938.

Rahman, B., Oliver, C. and Alderman, N. (2010). Descriptive functional analysis of challenging behaviours shown by adults with acquired brain injury. *Neuropsychological Rehabilitation, 20*, 212–238.

Tateno, A., Jage, R.E. and Robinson, R.G. (2003). Clinical correlates of aggressive behaviour after traumatic brain injury. *Journal of Neuropsychiatry and Clinical Neurosciences, 15*, 155–160.

Yudofsky, S.C., Silver, J.M., Jackson, W., Endicott, J. and Williams, D. (1986). The Overt Aggression Scale for the objective ratings of verbal and physical aggression. *American Journal of Psychiatry, 143*, 35–39.

Section III

Intervention

6 Neurobehavioural rehabilitation and application of new learning methods

Andrew Worthington and Nick Alderman

Introduction

This chapter will outline the practical techniques and their conceptual basis that form the principal means of intervention in neurobehavioural rehabilitation. Whilst these can be utilised in many therapeutic settings, it should be noted that NbR *services* provide environments that are specifically organised to optimise learning using these methods, while also providing a therapeutic milieu in which skills learned can be frequently practised in a social context until they (ideally) become habitual. A summary of the distinctive characteristics of how they are organised is described in Chapter 8 of this volume, and interested readers are referred to Wood, Alderman and Worthington (2020) for a detailed account of the historical development and contemporary characteristics of NbR services.

The causes of challenging behaviour after ABI are many and varied and have been discussed in Chapter 1. Although many factors can lead to challenging behaviour, in the context of ABI clinicians need to understand the nature of the brain injury in order to assess the likely contribution of the injury and to determine the most effective methods of learning (or re-learning) new skills.

Wood (1990) distinguished between three sources of behaviour disorder in cautioning that many professionals rush to 'manage' challenging behaviour without first considering its nature and the relationship to brain injury:

1 behaviour that is paroxysmal (described as 'electrically based') in the context of otherwise undisturbed behaviour, often accompanied by remorse;
2 behaviour associated with frontal brain injury characterised by irritability, short temper and low frustration tolerance with reduced self-control, leading to responses that escalate out of proportion to the trigger event;
3 wilful learned behaviour under conscious control, often threatening and used purposely for gratuitous reward.

These behavioural manifestations are not mutually exclusive and there may be multiple drivers to behaviour that evolve over time, hence it is important to consider a range of aetiologies. It would be equally remiss to attribute all

DOI: 10.4324/9781003083290-9

behaviour to brain injury and neglect pre- and post-morbid learning experiences, as that would be to ascribe all behaviour to the environment and ignore the underlying neuropsychological constraints on learning.

The field is constantly evolving. Some methods in early use are no longer considered acceptable, others remain mainstream, and new approaches are being developed as evidence accrues about the most effective forms of promoting behaviour change. An understanding of the underlying learning theory is essential for new methods must be grounded in established knowledge; reinforcement is not an opt-in for clinicians, they are either using it correctly or incorrectly (Worthington and Alderman, 2017); and, similarly, on a practical basis, Wood (1987) stated, 'senior staff must maintain constant vigilance to ensure that other members of staff project an atmosphere of encouragement, rather than allowing a sterile system of reinforcement to develop' (p. 55).

What follows is a concise summary of the range of evidence-based techniques at the clinician's disposal. In reviewing these interventions, we distinguish three broad approaches to changing behaviour: those based on changing the antecedent conditions (stimulus control), those based on changing the responses (response consequence) and those based on modifying self-control, potentially by recruiting internal cognitive mechanisms (self-regulation). It should be noted that these can be utilised to directly reduce challenging behaviours and to teach skills that fulfil the functions these serve, thus making them redundant.

Stimulus control techniques

Stimulus control methods are surprisingly commonplace in everyday life, underpinning many practical and social skills and are frequently used in therapy. They can be contrasted with contingency management approaches that manipulate the consequences of action in order to change behaviour (see below). Antecedent manipulations are based on the principle that the frequency of a behaviour can be reduced if the situations likely to provoke such behaviour can be identified. They form the basis for the development of positive behaviour support (PBS), an approach originally designed for people with a neurodevelopmental disability, which is distinguishable from behaviour support methods available from NbR, which was conceptualised to accommodate the different needs of people with ABI (see Chapter 7). Antecedent manipulations use a range of methods to increase the likelihood of adaptive behaviour, not least stimulus control. At its most basic, this involves recognising the relationship between an external event (the antecedent) and the behaviour (response). Relationships of this kind may be long-standing and natural, and can occur without conditioning. Thus, where the trigger event has an innate capacity to provoke a response (e.g., aggression in response to threat), it is known as an unconditioned stimulus and the behaviour as an unconditioned response, although prior learning experiences may also be relevant. Where the trigger event lacks an innate association and has to be learned (think of automatically pressing the brake pedal on approaching a red light) it is known as a conditional or conditioned stimulus and the behaviour is deemed a conditioned response. Although the precise mechanisms are still debated, the means by which an independent external event (the stimulus) becomes associated with an automatic response through repeated pairing is the essence of classical conditioning and forms the theoretical background to a range of practical interventions. Conditioning procedures of this nature can be used to tackle both maladaptive learned responses and powerful innately driven behavioural triggers that place people at risk of harm or social exclusion and that rehabilitation seeks to address. This is done either by reducing exposure to the trigger stimulus or by weakening the association between the stimulus and the undesirable response it provokes.

Environmental management

At its most basic, environmental management involves manipulating a person's immediate environment in order to eliminate salient aspects that act as triggers to challenging behaviour. This may be effective in reducing sensory overload – for example, a person who cannot tolerate a noisy dining room may take their meals at a different time or in a quiet area, thereby improving participation in rehabilitation (Slifer et al., 1997) and reducing social exclusion (Fluharty and Glassman, 2001). It may be sufficient to introduce an additional safeguard, for instance someone with an aversion to another vulnerable individual should not be left alone in their presence. Whilst having an intuitive appeal and often an immediate impact, evidence is largely anecdotal unless incorporated into a more comprehensive stimulus control programme. Although an important aspect of managing agitation in dementia (Wilkes et al., 2005), by itself environmental manipulation is often impractical, may have an adverse impact on others, is often a short-term solution only, does not address the underlying behaviour and does not promote new learning.

Discrimination training

In any setting the brain is bombarded by a multitude of events, famously described by William James in another context as a blooming, buzzing confusion of stimuli. That which has the most salience is likely to attract attention. Discrimination training seeks to address the shortfalls inherent in trying to change the environment rather than the person. Central to the implementation of stimulus control is the ability to discriminate between aspects of the environment in order to respond differentially to different setting conditions. It follows that learning can be enhanced by directing attention to particular events (rather than others). Yet simply exposing a person to a stimulus or cue does not guarantee the person will select that aspect of their environment as the most relevant. The aim of discrimination training is to maximise reinforcement by strengthening the association between a specific event and a desired response. This is a vitally important skill in everyday life as capacity for pro-social behaviour requires being able to distinguish social cues, initiating or inhibiting behaviour accordingly. As the ability to do so is often affected by ABI, it may be necessary to introduce a specific intervention for this purpose.

In one such scenario a specific stimulus is repeatedly presented (often over a matter of minutes) and a reinforcer is administered each time a desired response is observed, whilst no action is taken in the absence of the desired response. This establishes the link between stimulus and response. Stimulus discrimination is then introduced by interspersing another stimulus, any response to which is not reinforced; only the desired response to the original stimulus is followed by reinforcement. Once achieved, the ability of the person to respond only to the target stimulus is further improved by making the competing stimulus increasingly similar to this while maintaining reinforcement only for the former.

Alternatively, the target and competing stimuli can be presented at the same time, which theoretically may speed up learning as responding to the target stimulus inevitably involves not responding to the distractor stimulus. This latter method, whilst potentially helpful in overcoming severe memory impairment, may place greater demands on divided attention. Early studies by Wood (1987) show a correlation with results on tests of attention that suggests successive stimulus presentation may be the preferable method in circumventing attention deficits. Research indicates that attention control is a crucial mediator of sensory discrimination required for higher level cognitive function (Tsukahara et al., 2020). The clinician considering introducing a basic discrimination training, therefore, needs to consider the balance of attention and memory impairment when deciding to implement successive or simultaneous stimuli. In traumatic brain injury at least, where attention control deficits tend to predominate, the former may be preferable.

There is a wide variety of tasks that can be used as discrimination training incorporating stimuli of varying complexity. At a very basic level, of a kind that might be employed for people with sensory impairment or very severe cognitive deficits, it may be appropriate to address important perceptual discrimination. There is a key distinction, however, between the inability to make such a discrimination (e.g., due to apperceptive or associative agnosia) and the inability to respond appropriately, although the basis for the challenging behaviour may not be immediately apparent – in which case distinguishing between a behavioural and perceptual disorder may be the first stage of assessment. In some instances, behaviour becomes challenging due to problems with visual scanning or inattention, or because a person cannot make the necessary higher-level discrimination, which can affect appraisal of stimuli as diverse as foodstuffs and facial expression. An early example involved training a woman to recognise visuospatial cues in order to position her wheelchair correctly to execute safe transfers (Wood, 1988). In other cases, perceptual recognition is clearly intact and, in the context of poor inhibitory control, drives the challenging behaviour (utilisation behaviour is a stark example of such stimulus-driven action).

Shaping

In any process of skill acquisition, it takes time to execute an action smoothly and efficiently and the process of learning is one of gradually honing one's efforts until eventually the desired level of competence is achieved. Shaping involves the reinforcement of successive approximations to a desired target behaviour. Training someone to self-feed, for example, may involve reinforcing what might be initially a rather random action of grasping a spoon; once spoon grasping has been accomplished, reinforcement shifts towards moving the spoon towards the mouth and subsequently for inserting spoon in the mouth. In this way an exploratory or otherwise random behaviour is gradually shaped towards a purposeful action, which becomes self-sustaining by its own intrinsic reinforcement value of obtaining food. Shaping utilises discriminative learning because, as Wood (1990, p. 159) stated, 'as the process of reinforcing [successive] approximations proceeds, responses which are increasingly similar to the final goal are reinforced while those responses dissimilar to the final goal are not reinforced, the former increasing, the latter decreasing.'

Thus, shaping is a method of changing behaviour and may initially involve reinforcing behaviour far removed from the eventual objective. This is in contrast to chaining discussed below in which each small behavioural step learned early in the procedure remains intact as part of the overall behavioural outcome.

Chaining

Unlike shaping, chaining reinforces existing behaviours that are effective components of a series of actions towards a goal. In contrast with shaping, which always proceeds in a forwards direction, chaining can proceed forwards or backwards (in the latter case commencing with the final step in a sequence). Chaining is a useful method for developing complex behaviours that can be broken down into smaller steps, on the basis that it is easier to learn a single action than a sequence of actions. As most therapy activities involve a series of actions to achieve a functional goal, chaining offers a means of assisting people to focus on the building blocks of a complex behaviour in a series of steps. The initial therapy goal becomes the attainment of an individual step in a multi-step sequence rather than the complete sequence. The therapist first has to determine how many subgoals a task should be divided into. For example, the task of 'getting ready for the day'. For on person it may be sufficient to divide this into three stages such as:

1 Getting out of bed
2 Getting washed
3 Getting dressed.

However, another person may require the task to be divided into more steps, perhaps because the ability to learn is undermined by serious neurocognitive impairment, as follows:

1 Getting out of bed
2 Walking to bathroom
3 Turning on water in shower
4 Checking water temperature

5 Getting into shower
6 Putting shampoo on hair
7 Washing hair
8 Rinsing hair

An observational assessment is required to determine the appropriate number of steps that will reflect the level of action complexity a person can execute unaided. As their behaviour will also be influenced by their physical status, a range of motor and sensory difficulties may need to be taken into account in determining both the level of task breakdown and the nature of prompting.

The essence of chaining is that completion of one stage acts as a prompt (discriminative stimulus) for the next step in the sequence. Initially this may require a verbal or physical prompt by the therapist in order to move to the next step. Forward chaining starts at the beginning of a task and proceeds through to completion as in the steps described above. Backward chaining may be more effective in severe cases, however, which is a procedure where the therapist undertakes or assists with all but the final step to allow this to be completed independently. Once this is executed satisfactorily the therapist completes all but the last two steps and works progressively backwards through the sequence. Over time, in both forward and backward chaining, the sequence becomes ingrained by repetition. In performing complex actions, it can be useful to ask the person to repeat a verbal prompt because this provides additional reinforcement by linking language with action and paves the way for self-prompting in the absence of a therapist (see section on self-regulation below).

Chaining is often described in terms of its application to temporal sequences of behaviour in a specific location (e.g., a bedroom or a kitchen), but it can also be used for spatial sequencing. The first author has also used this method for training way-finding, from the ability to locate a bedroom in a rehabilitation facility to being able to visit a local shop independently. Figure 6.1 depicts a hypothetical route a person might need to learn in a rehabilitation facility from their bedroom (marked as A) to the garden (located at E). In forward chaining,

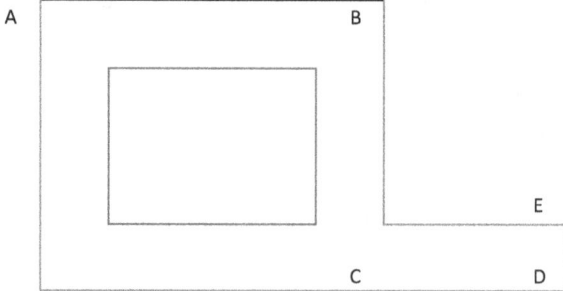

Figure 6.1 Chaining programme to assist getting from bedroom (A) to garden (E) in rehabilitation centre allows forward chaining (A–B–C–D–E) or backward chaining (E–D–C–B–A).

the sequence begins by prompting the person how to get from A to B and proceeds from there on the basis that once they were at B they would know how to get to C from where they could locate D and thereafter find E. In backward chaining, a person would be taken as far as D and asked to get to E independently. Once they had shown they could get to E from D, they would be taken from A as far as C and asked to complete C–D–E independently, and so on until they could start from A and compete the full route.

Errorless learning

Backward chaining may be particularly helpful because it maximises the opportunity for reinforcement early in the intervention. In Figure 6.1, it is only necessary to go from D to E independently to achieve the goal, and only once that has been achieved reliably, does the task become a little more challenging with reinforcement now based on getting from C to E autonomously. In essence this is a form of errorless learning because the next phase of the intervention (going from C to E instead of from D to E) is only introduced once the previous step is learned, so effectively a person only has to learn to get from C to D because once at D they know how to locate E.

Initially introduced to assist people with severe anterograde amnesia, errorless learning was shown to be superior to trial-and-error learning (Wilson et al., 1994). Although not without its critics – Middleton and Schwartz (2012), for example, argued that the benefits had been overstated – errorless learning methods have been utilised in training life skills (Cohen et al., 2010), as a means of optimising other techniques such as goal management training (Bertens et al., 2015) and, as the example above illustrates, can be utilised for a range of tasks including way-finding as well verbal and motor tasks.

Response consequence learning

Response consequence learning is based on the principles of instrumental or operant learning. Manipulating the consequences of behaviour to change the behaviour itself was an early development of the classical conditioning paradigm. In both scenarios, a stimulus A is followed by a significant event B but, whereas in classical conditioning both events occurred outside the agency of the individual organism, instrumental conditioning takes place as a result of the individual learning to perform action A in order to bring out the desired outcome B. In NbR, this involves delivering reinforcement B upon occurrence of behaviour A but not after behaviour A<prime> in order to increase the probability that A will occur more often than A<prime> or any other undesired or irrelevant action. Referring to the benefits of this approach within the conventional distinction of antecedents–behaviour–consequences (ABC analysis), Eames (1988) stated, 'we are not, in fact, able to be in control of "antecedents" in the real world, yet success in any kind of rehabilitation means being accepted in that real world. So in order to be sufficiently controlled in behaviour, the person is going to have to put up with all sorts of "A"s' (p. 52). This is supported by a more recent literature review of interventions to improve engagement in rehabilitation suggesting that contingency management approaches are the most effective (Brett, Sykes and Pires-Yfantouda, 2017).

Time-out

All interactions have a reinforcement potential, meaning that a response to a behaviour is either likely to increase or decrease the probability of recurrence. In order to avoid increasing the likelihood of an undesirable behaviour, it may be necessary to withdraw attention that might unwittingly be positively reinforcing. Time-out from positive reinforcement ('time-out' for short) is a therapeutic tool intended to avoid such consequences by removing potential reinforcements for a brief period of time. In this way a person learns certain actions do not result in favourable outcomes. One means of doing this is to guide a person away from the situation in order to remove them from sources of reinforcement. This is done with the minimum of engagement, to avoid unwittingly reinforcing the behaviour, and is sometimes augmented by a cue-word to develop the association between the behaviour and the response. Somewhat paradoxically, Stewart and Alderman (2010) showed that situational time-out could be effective in reducing behaviour reinforced by escape-avoidance because of the opportunity it provided for a brief respite from the antecedent trigger and was always followed by re-exposure to the original task. The authors reported a marked reduction in aggression during personal hygiene routines after just 12 sessions.

Sometimes it can be difficult to encourage someone away from a situation without escalating their behaviour. The technique of 'time-out-on-the-spot from positive reinforcement' (TOOTS for short) can be a very effective means of withholding reinforcement; it may involve the clinician or carer walking away briefly (without giving any indication they are affected by the behaviour) or remaining in situ and refraining from any action (such as conversation or eye contact) that could be reinforcing. A response of this nature may be counterintuitive and can be difficult to sustain, but is only necessary for brief periods, sometimes of just a few seconds, to be effective before re-engaging. Of course, this assumes the person is normally in receipt of social reinforcement, otherwise it is impossible to time-out, as Eames (1988) put it, 'if you are usually ignored, then you are unlikely to notice being ignored' (p. 53).

Worthington and Wood (2009) reported the case of RB, a 29-year-old clerical worker who sustained severe brain injury resulting in dysexecutive disorder, labile mood, poor social communication skills, and disinhibited behaviour, including persistent spitting and ritualised toilet behaviours. After unsuccessful efforts to manage his behaviour in the community, RB was admitted to a residential neurobehavioural facility where he received a range of interventions including TOOTS for spitting. Staff were instructed to initiate social contact with RB whenever he was observed without spitting and trained to briefly disengage for 30 seconds when he began to spit, re-engaging after this time if he had ceased spitting. By using this TOOTS method he was reinforced for not spitting. After 12 weeks spitting had reduced by almost 70% which meant that social interactions persisted for longer and were more intrinsically rewarding, thereby helping to maintain the treatment gains.

Extinction

Extinction refers to the process by which a behaviour gradually ceases to be associated with a specific antecedent due to the absence of reinforcement. A classic paradigm in animal studies would be to fail to provide the food whose arrival an animal had previously learned was heralded by a stimulus like a light or buzzer. The animal would eventually stop salivating in response to the signal. How does this translate to brain injury rehabilitation? Essentially extinction is a process of *un*learning a behaviour; the frequency is either reduced or eliminated altogether by breaking (unlearning) the link between a response and its trigger stimulus. For this purpose, the technique of response prevention (for example with enuresis, nail-biting or thumb-sucking) has some empirical support (van Houten and Rolider, 1984; Luciano et al., 1993). Response prevention was a component of treatment for inappropriate sexual behaviour in an adolescent with intellectual disability reported by Shenk and Brown (2007). It is usually only one aspect of a broad range of treatment methods, however it can be difficult to implement and raises ethical concerns. Alternatively, desensitisation procedures may be effective in addressing habitual behaviours and can be utilised in graded fashion (e.g., Youngson and Alderman, 1994), which is advisable in brain injury rather than using flooding/implosion methods due to the frequency of emotional dysregulation after ABI.

Extinction methods seek to extinguish undesirable behaviour by reducing the effectiveness of reinforcers maintaining them. In some instances, this is achieved though repeated presentation of an antecedent trigger stimulus leading to satiation. In an early psychiatric case that has since become rather celebrated, a long-term hospitalised patient who hoarded multiple towels daily in her room (between 19 and 29) was not only allowed to keep the towels (in contrast to previous staff responses) but provided with additional towels by staff without any comment, starting at 7 additional towels per day and increasing to as many as 60 a day, with the patient stating after two weeks she did not need any more towels and by the sixth week of intervention she was removing the towels herself, gains that persisted through the six-month follow-up phase (Allyon, 1963).

Alternatively, multiple repetitions of the target behaviour (negative practice) may also lead to a reduced frequency of the behaviour outside the intervention session. This probably weakens the reinforcement value of the behaviour and may increase response inhibition as a result of fatigue (reactive inhibition). The aversive fatigue-related inhibition dissipates once the behaviour ceases, resulting in cessation being negatively reinforced. Noting that extinction-based or reward programmes often failed to address escape-avoidance behaviours, Alderman

(1991) used satiation through negative practice to reduce the frequency and duration of prolonged shouting in a severely brain-injured adult, enabling physical and functional gains to be achieved through increased participation in rehabilitation. There is no set duration or frequency of negative practice, studies outside the brain injury field ranging from a minute to an hour, and clinicians must determine the issue on a case-by-case basis. Lewis et al. (1986) found no difference between 15 seconds and 1 minute of negative practice in self-stimulatory leg-pounding in a brain-injured adult, as both were equally effective in reducing the behaviour in sessions but neither led to generalised improvement outside the sessions. In such cases it is necessary to broaden the scope of intervention to incorporate other contexts by way of generalisation training.

Differential reinforcement

There are many clinical situations where in order to reduce or extinguish one behaviour it is necessary or desirable to promote a substitute behaviour. Differential reinforcement is helpful when a person is capable of a range of behaviours and the therapist wishes to modify their probability of occurrence, differentiating between behaviour to be encouraged and that to be discouraged. It differs from discrimination training in that discrimination training seeks to improve awareness of salient aspects of the environment whereas differential reinforcement methods aim increase the frequency of behaviour being exhibited. Differential reinforcement programmes are characterised by prescribing different responses to different behaviours, often referred to as differential reinforcement of other behaviour (DRO) programmes. For example, if the target behaviour to be reduced is non-compliance or shouting, a fixed-interval reinforcement schedule is established and reinforcement is provided after each interval within which the behaviour is absent. This is a well-established technique and is often a method of choice where certain behaviours have become inadvertently reinforced. This can be effective even if the target behaviour occurs much less frequently than the inappropriate behaviour, but the interval needs to be appropriate to the frequency of the behaviour. A very high frequency of behaviour may mean the person never achieves the reward, in which case a DRL procedure would be more appropriate (see below).

DRO methods have been used successfully in addressing instances of self-injurious acts. Hefferman and Lyons (2016) introduced a DRO programme in response to habitual nail-biting, for example. Partial-interval recording was used to establish a baseline with two therapists achieving a reliability of 92 per cent for their baseline observations. Nail-biting occurred on average 38 times per session. Access to a tactile reinforcer was contingent on refraining from nail-biting during a specified time interval. This was initially set at 20 seconds to allow multiple opportunities for reward, using a visible timer that would be reset if nail-biting occurred during the interval. Over time, the duration of the DRO interval was increased and once it reached 60 minutes was removed with reinforcers being introduced into the natural environment.

Often it is desirable to reinforce a specific alternative response. Hollon (1972) introduced a programme to selectively reinforce cooperative and self-care actions that were incompatible with disruptive behaviours that had unwittingly been reinforced and that were undermining rehabilitation in the community. A person might be reinforced, for example, by keeping their arm extended when walking rather than using a habitual flexed position. As performance of the behaviour to be reinforced often prevents execution of the inappropriate behaviour, they are sometimes referred to as differential reinforcement of incompatible behaviour (DRI) programmes.

With very high frequency, behaviours limiting reinforcement to the absence of a target behaviour interval may not be feasible and instead a target threshold is set below the baseline frequency. This is known as differential reinforcement of low rates of behaviour (DRL), the threshold set for reinforcement gradually reducing over time. Alderman and Knight (1997) demonstrated a range of advantages that DRL interventions have over DRO/DRI procedures. They reported successful use of DRL in managing challenging behaviour in three cases with follow-up data up to 18 months post-treatment.

Watson et al. (2001) reported the case of JH, whose aggression was successfully reduced 10 years after sustaining a gunshot wound to the brain using DRL. The day was divided into four equal time-periods and JH was given a star as a reward at the end of each period for which the frequency of his aggression was below a threshold. The highest level of aggressive incidents recorded was 55 and it was considered likely he would be able to achieve a reward contingent on a threshold of 18 aggressive incidents per time-period initially. If JH was successful in obtaining the reward, he would be given profuse social praise and helped to fix the star on to a wall chart, otherwise the reason why he did not achieve a star was explained and he was reminded there would be a further opportunity within the next time-period. At the end of each day, he was informed how many stars he had achieved and, once he obtained all four, these could be exchanged for a tangible reward or 'banked' for a more substantial reinforcer. Over the 85-week intervention period the threshold was gradually reduced until it was set at just two incidents of aggression and accompanied by a reduction in antipsychotic medication. The widespread use of tangible reinforcers characterised the token economies of many psychiatric, forensic and learning disability institutions of the past and were instrumental in early efforts to address challenging behaviour in ABI (Eames and Wood, 1985) but are now more often encountered in circumscribed fashion rather than systemically – for example, Manchester (1997) in reducing absconding from a rehabilitation ward.

Response-cost

Neurocognitive impairment can undermine successful learning using the above methods. For example, Alderman (1996) proffered experimental evidence that demonstrated that the presence of severe difficulties with memory and the allocation of attentional resources prevented engagement in behaviour support plans that utilised positive reinforcement and extinction principles. However, use of a further operant learning paradigm, that of response-cost, provides a means that enables effective learning in spite of these impairments, including severe anterograde amnesia (Alderman and Burgess, 1994). See Chapter 9 for an example of use of response-cost.

A final comment in this section should address the use of non-contingent reinforcement (NCR), which contrasts with other approaches reviewed above as reinforcement such as social attention is delivered for a specified period regardless of the behaviour. This method is proposed in response to criticisms of differential reinforcement. It comprises three phases: (i) fixed time-interval reinforcement; (ii) extinction with no response to target behaviour; and (iii) fading out reinforcement. It has been widely used in treatment of self-injurious behaviour as an alternative to DRO and is particularly effective where the non-contingent reinforcement matches the function of the challenging behaviour (Vollmer et al., 1993; Persel et al., 1997).

Self-regulation methods

The evolution of neurobehavioural methods from conditioning-based procedures to techniques aimed to improve self-regulation has many threads, among which social learning theory and neuropsychological models of cognition have been central (see Worthington and Alderman, 2017).

Even the arch-behaviourist Skinner (1973), whilst considering that awareness could be better understood within the language of reinforcement, recognised the potential therapeutic value of this approach: 'Awareness may help if the problem is in part a lack of awareness, and "insight" into one's condition may help if one then takes remedial action' (p. 188). Unfortunately, in ABI impairments of selective attention and working memory can undermine conventional conditioning-based approaches and executive deficiencies in judgement, decision making and initiative mean that an intellectual level of awareness does not readily translate into compensatory action. Fortunately, the importance of language in regulating behaviour (notions traceable to Vygotsky and Luria) provides a rationale in utilising language to address challenging behaviour. Early developmental work showing that impulsive and aggressive children used language differently led to efforts to train skills of verbal mediation (thinking out loud), combining self-instruction with operant learning theory by increasing self-observation and addressing maladaptive behaviour with incompatible verbal prompts (Meichenbaum, 1977). Seeking to integrate problem-solving insights into behaviour modification, D'zurilla and Goldfried (1971) developed a form of self-control that highlighted important stages of goal orientation and problem definition, generation of alternatives, decision making and verification, a forerunner of goal management training.

Self-regulation methods can take many forms of varying cognitive demands with the overriding objective of promoting pro-social and adaptive behaviour through self-control and self-initiation. Cognitive constraints on attention and memory, however, may compromise their success. Matthey (1996) employed verbal feedback in an attempt to improve self-monitoring to reduce the frequency of an anoxic woman's persistent requests to telephone home with temporary success, but it became necessary to disconnect the phone for 30 seconds outside of her allotted two calls per day in order to extinguish the behaviour.

Alderman, Fry and Youngson (1995) developed a self-monitoring training (SMT) intervention to address some of the limitations in response-cost, including generalisability. This focused first on developing awareness of specific behaviours in order to facilitate reductions of the target behaviour in a DRL procedure. In a subsequent study, Knight et al. (2002) suggested that incorporating a self-monitoring element to differential reinforcement may result in longer but more sustained learning. Evidence of spontaneous generalisability was described by Worthington (2005) in addressing disinhibited speech in a young woman following encephalitis and by Dayus and van den Broek (2000) in reducing delusion confabulations.

Bandura's (1977) notion that learning proceeds by expectation of reinforcement (by which beliefs about schedules of reinforcement and their attainment can exert greater influence on behaviour than the reinforcement itself) suggests that improving self-efficacy is an effective way of changing behaviour. Self-mastery was included in an intervention to reduce anxiety and shouting during personal care by providing instruction on using shower controls and a set spoken phrase considered to aid with cognitive restructuring (Burgess and Alderman, 1990). Zenicus and colleagues (1990) incorporated self-monitoring, feedback and skills training to address hypersexual behaviour after frontal brain injury (Study II). Self-regulation approaches also embrace some of the skills-based methods characteristic of positive behaviour programming by promoting functional and coping skills in the form of modified cognitive schema, as in the case of Burgess and Alderman (1990) described above.

Conclusion

This chapter has reviewed the practical techniques and their conceptual basis for the most common types of intervention in NbR. While the scientific literature (and some practitioners) maintains a distinct division between antecedent or stimulus control methods and contingency management approaches, in practice the complexity of challenging behaviour after ABI means that effective interventions frequently have multiple components (e.g., Rothwell, LaVigna and Willis 1999). The chapter emphasis has been on those methods that have been shown to be efficacious in learning new or alternative behaviours, as this is the most effective way to reduce challenging and disruptive behaviour and also the most acceptable form of NbR today. Even where there is a need to reduce a behaviour because of the potential for harm and the resulting level of disability and social exclusion, focusing solely on elimination is likely to be less effective as a general principle than aiming to replace maladaptive behaviour with an alternative more productive and less stigmatising behaviour. There will always be a need for creative solutions to challenging behaviour, but practitioners have the benefit of decades of clinical research and innovation and a strong evidence base to inform their design and implementation of neurobehavioural interventions.

References

Alderman, N. (1991). The treatment of avoidance behaviour following severe brain injury by satiation through negative practice. *Brian Injury, 5* (1), 77–86.

Alderman, N. (1996). Central executive deficit and response cost operant conditioning methods. *Neuropsychological Rehabilitation, 6,* 161–186.

Alderman, N. and Burgess, P. (1994). A comparison of treatment methods for behaviour disorders following herpes simplex encephalitis. *Neuropsychological Rehabilitation, 4,* 31–48.

Alderman, N., Fry, R. and Youngson, H. (1995). Improvement of self-monitoring skills, reduction of behaviour disturbance and the dysexecutive syndrome: Comparison of response cost and a new programme of self-monitoring training. *Neuropsychological Rehabilitation, 5* (3), 193–221.

Alderman, N. and Knight, C. (1997). Effectiveness of DRL in the management and treatment of severe behaviour disorders following brain injury. *Brain Injury, 11* (2), 79–102.

Allyon, T. (1963). Intensive treatment of psychotic behaviour by stimulus satiation and food reinforcement. *Behaviour Research and Therapy, 1,* 53–62.

Bandura, A. (1977). Self-efficacy: Toward a unifying theory of behavioural change. *Psychological Review, 84* (2), 191–215.

Bertens, D., Kessels, R., Fiorenzato, E., Boelen, D. and Fasotti, L. (2015). Do old errors always lead to new truths? A randomized controlled trial of errorless goal management training in brain-injured patients. *Journal of the International Neuropsychological Society, 21* (8), 639–649.

Brett, C.E., Sykes, C. and Pires-Yfantouda, R. (2017). Interventions to increase engagement with rehabilitation in adults with acquired brain injury: A systematic review. *Neuropsychological Rehabilitation, 27* (9), 959–982.

Burgess, P.W. and Alderman, N. (1990). Rehabilitation of dyscontrol syndromes following frontal lobe damage: A cognitive neuropsychological approach. In R.Ll. Wood and I. Fussey (eds), *Cognitive Rehabilitation in Perspective* (pp. 183–203). London: Taylor and Francis.

Cohen, M., Ylvisaker, M., Hamilton, J., Kemp, L. and Claiman, B. (2010). Errorless learning of functional life skills in an individual with three aetiologies of severe memory and executive function impairment. *Neuropsychological Rehabilitation, 20* (3), 355–376.

Dayus, B. and van den Broek, M. (2000). Treatment of stable delusional confabulations using self-monitoring training. *Neuropsychological Rehabilitation, 10* (4), 415–427.

D'Zurilla, T.J., and Goldfried, M.R. (1971). Problem solving and behavior modification. *Journal of Abnormal Psychology, 78* (1), 107–126.

Eames, P. (1988). Some aspects of the management of difficult behaviour. In P. Hall and P.D. Stonier (eds), *Perspectives in Psychiatry: The Worcester Lectures* (pp. 41–58). London: John Wiley and Sons.

Eames, P. and Wood, R.Ll. (1985). Rehabilitation after severe brain injury: A follow-up of a behaviour modification approach. *Journal of Neurology, Neurosurgery and Psychiatry, 48,* 613–619.

Fluharty, G. and Glassman, N. (2001). Use of antecedent control to improve the outcome of rehabilitation for a client with frontal lobe injury and intolerance for auditory and tactile stimuli. *Brain Injury, 15* (201), 995–1002.

Hefferman, L. and Lyons, D. (2016). Differential reinforcement of other behaviour for the reduction of severe nail biting. *Behaviour Analysis Practice, 9*, 253–256.

Hollon, T.H. (1972). Behaviour modification in a community hospital rehabilitation unit. *Archives of Physical Medicine and Rehabilitation, 54*, 65–68.

Knight, C., Rutterford, N.A. Alderman, N. and Swan, L.J. (2002). Is accurate self-monitoring necessary for people with acquired neurological problems to benefit from the use of differential reinforcement methods? *Brain Injury, 16* (1), 75–87.

Lewis, F.D., Blackerby, W.F., Ross, J.R., Guth, M. L., Cronkey, R.F., White, M.J. and Cook, T. (1986). *Behavioral Residential Treatment, 1* (4), 265–274.

Luciano, M.C., Molina, F.J., Gomez, I. and Herruzo, J. (1993). Response prevention and contingency management in the treatment of nocturnal neurosis. *Child and Family Behavior Therapy, 15* (1), 37–51.

Manchester, D. (1997). A non-aversive approach to reducing hospital absconding in a head-injured adolescent boy. *Brain Injury, 11* (4), 271–277.

Matthey, S. (1996). Modification of perseverative behaviour in an adult with anoxic brain damage. *Brain Injury, 10* (3), 219–227.

Meichenbaum, D. (1977). *Cognitive-Behaviour Modification. An Integrative Approach.* New York: Plenum Press.

Middleton, E.L. and Schwartz, M.F. (2012). Errorless learning in cognitive rehabilitation: A critical review. *Neuropsychological Rehabilitation, 22* (2), 138–168.

Persel, C.S., Persel, C.H., Ashley, M.J. and Krych, D.K., (1997). The use of noncontingent reinforcement and contingent restraint to reduce physical aggression and self-injurious behaviour in a traumatically brain-injured adult. *Brain Injury, 11* (10), 751–760.

Rothwell, N.A., LaVigna, G.W. and Willis, T.J. (1999). A nonaversive rehabilitation approach for people with severe behavioural problems resulting from brain injury. *Brain Injury, 13*, 521–533.

Shenk, C. and Brown, A. (2007). Cognitive-behavioural treatment of an adolescent sexual offender with an intellectual disability. *Clinical Case Studies, 6* (4), 307–324.

Skinner, B.F. (1973). *Beyond Freedom and Dignity.* Harmondsworth: Pelican Books.

Slifer, K., Tucker, C.L., Gerson, A.C., Sevier, R.C., Kane, A.C., Amari, A. and Clawson, B.P. (1997). Antecedent management and compliance training improve adolescents' participation in early brain injury rehabilitation. *Brain Injury, 11* (12), 877–890.

Stewart, I. and Alderman, N. (2010). Active versus passive management of post-acquired brain injury challenging behaviour: A case study analysis of multiple operant procedures in the treatment of challenging behaviour maintained by negative reinforcement. *Brain Injury, 24* (13–14), 1616–1627.

Tsukahara, J.S., Harison, T.L., Draheim, C., Martin, J.D. and Engle, R.W. (2020). Attention control: The missing link between sensory discrimination and intelligence. *Attention, Perception and Psychophysics, 82*, 3445–3478.

Van Houten, R. and Rolider, A. (1984). The use of response prevention to eliminate nocturnal thumbsucking. *Journal of Applied Behavior Analysis, 17* (4), 509–520.

Vollmer, T.R., Iwata, B.A., Zarcone, J.R., Smith, R.G. and Mazaleski, J.L. (1993). The role of attention in the treatment of attention-maintained self-injurious behavior: Noncontingent reinforcement and differential reinforcement of other behaviour. *Journal of Applied Behavior Analysis, 26*, 9–21.

Watson, C., Rutterford, N.A., Shortland, D., Williamson, N. and Alderman, N. (2001). Reduction of chronic aggressive behaviour 10 years after brain injury. *Brain Injury*, *15* (11), 1003–1015.

Wilkes, L., Fleming, A., Wilkes, B.L., Cioffi, J.M. and Le Miere, J. (2005). Environmental approach to reducing agitation in older persons with dementia in a nursing home. *Australasian Journal on Ageing*, *24* (3), 141–145.

Wilson, B.A., Baddeley, A., Evans, J. and Shiel, A. (1994). Errorless learning in the rehabilitation of memory impaired people. *Neuropsychological Rehabilitation*, *4* (3), 307–326.

Wood, R.Ll. (1987). *Brain Injury Rehabilitation: A Neurobehavioural Approach*. London: Croom Helm

Wood, R.Ll. (1988). Management of behaviour disorders in a day treatment setting. *Journal of Head Trauma Rehabilitation*, *3* (3), 53–62.

Wood, R.Ll. (1990). Conditioning procedures in brain injury rehabilitation. In R.Ll. Wood (ed.), *Neurobehavioural Sequelae of Traumatic Brain Injury* (pp. 153–174). London: Taylor and Francis.

Wood, R.Ll., Alderman, N. and Worthington, A. (2020). Neurobehavioural rehabilitation. In N. Agrawal, R. Faruqui and M. Bodani (eds), *Oxford Textbook of Neuropsychiatry* (pp. 475–481). Oxford: Oxford University Press.

Worthington, A. (2005). Rehabilitation of executive deficits: Effective treatment of related disabilities. In P. Halligan and D.T. Wade (eds), *Effectiveness of Rehabilitation for Cognitive Deficits* (pp. 257). New York: Oxford University Press.

Worthington, A. and Alderman, N. (2017). Neurobehavioural rehabilitation: A developing paradigm. In T.M. McMillan and R.Ll. Wood (eds), *Neurobehavioural Disability and Social Handicap Following Traumatic Brain Injury* (2nd edn) (pp. 15–29). New York: Routledge.

Worthington, A. and Wood, R.Ll. (2009). Behaviour problems. In A. Tyerman and N.S. King (eds), *Psychological Approaches to Rehabilitation After Traumatic Brain Injury* (pp. 228–259). Oxford: BPS Blackwell.

Youngson, H. and Alderman, N. (1994). Fear of incontinence and its effect on a community-based rehabilitation programme after severe brain injury: Successful remediation of escape behaviour using behaviour modification. *Brain Injury*, *8* (1), 23–36.

Zencius, A., Wesolowksi, M.D., Burke, W. and Hough, S. (1990). Managing hypersexual disorders in brain-injured clients. *Brain Injury*, *4* (2), 175–181.

7 Behaviour support in the context of neurobehavioural rehabilitation

Paul Mooney, Jenny Brooks and Niall Diggin

The impact of acquired brain injury

The impact of ABI can be devastating, leading to a range of life-changing difficulties for the individual, as well as those in their social circle. While the effects of ABI are unique to the person, they may include difficulties across multiple domains, including physical, emotional, cognitive and behavioural. Specific to neurobehavioural disability, it is often reported that individuals experience executive and attentional dysfunctions, alongside personality change, alexithymia, lability of mood and deficits in impulse control and insight (Williams et al., 2020; Alderman and Wood, 2013).

Damage to areas of the brain such as the orbitofrontal cortex (Morgan and Lilienfeld, 2000), temporal lobe (Tonkonogy, 1991) and prefrontal cortex (Siever, 2008) have been implicated in the development of challenging behaviour. Injury to such areas may reduce a person's ability to regulate their behaviour effectively, to make effective decisions and to plan ahead, which can in turn impact on multiple domains of that person's life and, in the extreme, can lead to contact with the criminal justice system and/or require the need for formal treatment. The primary focus of NbR is to develop an understanding of challenging behaviour and to provide interventions based on psychological theories that seek to reduce its frequency and intensity and to support regulation and/or habituation of behaviour.

Defining challenging behaviour

In the context of ABI, challenging behaviour can take many forms, and without intervention can endure or increase in frequency and intensity over time, even after the person regains functional and cognitive skills (Alderman, 2001). Typically, verbal and physical aggression have been cited as the most common forms of challenging behaviour observed in this population. However, it is also common to observe poor motivation/low arousal, non-cooperation, self-harm, sexual inappropriateness and other behaviours that may serve to exclude the person from some services, therapies or, indeed, from society.

DOI: 10.4324/9781003083290-10

Of course, not all who suffer a brain injury experience disturbance of behaviour, however research has suggested it is a significant possibility. In a study by Visscher et al. (2011), 42 per cent of patients in a neuropsychiatric ward engaged in one or more aggressive behaviours, with a smaller number of patients (14 per cent) being responsible for the majority of incidents (70 per cent). Rao et al. (2009) reported that the prevalence of aggressive behaviour in their sample of 67 participants with first-time ABI was 28.4 per cent, and this was predominantly verbal aggression rather than physical. When considering those engaged in NbR, Alderman, Knight and Henman (2002) reported that during a 14-day period, 46 patients exhibited 3,914 acts of aggression. Similar to the study by Rao et al. (2009), most acts of aggression were verbal, but still with a significant number of acts of physical aggression ($n = 443$) recorded during this period. As such, it can be concluded that individuals with ABI can experience problems with disturbed behaviour, with those admitted to NbR services exhibiting a more significant frequency and, arguably, intensity of such behaviours.

Restrictive practice

Restrictive practices are efforts to manage challenging behaviour that, by definition, restrict the freedom and choice of an individual at times of significant risk of harm. Such interventions include the use of restraint, seclusion and rapid tranquilisation. There has been considerable focus on the use of such restrictive interventions for many years in the wake of high-profile deaths and scandals involving the abuse and neglect of patients in psychiatric services (e.g., Winterbourne View, South Gloucestershire), where restriction became embedded in daily clinical practice, rather than being used sparingly, as a last resort.

The use of physical restraint in the management of psychiatric patients has a history dating back at least 300 years. Historically, a lack of governing body to oversee the use of restraint techniques and a lack of training had led to many patients and staff being harmed. The use of both mechanical and physical restraint continues, although the regulation of such practices has improved considerably. Such improvements have at times been driven by high-profile deaths in inpatient services where inappropriate techniques were being utilised or where the physical health needs of the patient had not been taken into consideration. Despite the ethical concerns about the use of restraint, however, it remains a necessary component of these services, as a means of enhancing the safety of patients and staff, so long as, of course, it is monitored and regulated effectively.

In addition to restraint, medication has been used to subdue patients exhibiting heightened aggression, but historically this restrictive intervention has led to some patients being over-sedated. While this can lead to a reduction in challenging behaviour, it is an artificial solution that can be ineffective as a longer-term strategy. Whilst the use of medication to provide short-term management of behaviour can provide enhanced safety in acute situations, arguably it can interfere with the person's ability to learn; and given that NbR is largely based upon learning theories, this may be problematic in some cases. Also, an over-reliance on medication to manage challenging behaviour may signify a lack of behaviour support initiatives (in the form of supporting new learning and the provision of behavioural interventions).

History of behaviour support

A central component of many types of clinical provision, whether inpatient or community services, is that of the management of challenging behaviour, or 'behaviour support'. As such, the service goal is to reduce or extinguish the challenging behaviour so that the person can integrate back into society; or, if the behaviour is considered to be a barrier to treatment, to reduce it to the extent that the person can engage meaningfully. Either way, being able to effectively describe and implement behaviour support is critical to most service types.

Over the years, there have been various approaches to behaviour support, although arguably most are to some extent rooted in the behaviourist tradition. At the time of writing, the most widely known approach is that of 'positive behavioural support', which is most commonly associated with the support of people with neurodevelopmental disorders. However, PBS is not the only documented method of behaviour support, although there are significant overlaps in philosophy and approach.

Behaviour therapy originated as far back as the early 1900s, but became more established as a formal psychological approach during the 1950s, when it referenced to the application of interventions based upon learning principles (Larkin and Zvolensky, 2001). The work of behaviour support that we see today is largely based on the efforts of influential experimental psychologists such as Pavlov, Watson, Skinner and Bandura. Their work highlighted the idea that behaviour was largely shaped by a person's environment, by watching and copying the behaviour of others, and through other forms of learning. As such, learning theories play a central part in how we understand the developmental trajectory of both pro-social and challenging behaviour and, as such, they underpin many of the behaviour support strategies utilised in NbR services.

The term 'positive behavioural support' describes a broad approach that outlines how clinicians can manage the various physical, social, educational and logistical support structures needed to achieve basic lifestyle goals while reducing problem behaviours that pose barriers to these goals (Dunlap et al., 2009; Dunlap and Carr, 2007; Koegel, Koegel and Dunlap, 1996). Specifically, PBS is a framework recommended for use in neurodevelopmental populations, where clients may have diagnoses of learning disability and/or autism, although the adoption of PBS plans (or the equivalent) that advise staff how to support the person is advised across all service types by the UK Mental Health Act (1983; revised 2007).

PBS is a central focus for those clients with neurodevelopmental disorders, and is often framed as a multi-dimensional, person-centred framework that seeks to improve the quality of life for an individual, as well as supporting them in learning new skills and adapt their physical environments to meet sensory needs. As such, challenging behaviour for people with learning disability or autism is often seen to be the result of a reduced quality of life, with the assumption that an improvement in their quality of life will lead to a reduction of the challenging behaviour itself. However, in ABI populations, quality of life in itself may be an insufficient treatment target, given the nature of most brain injuries.

While PBS is the framework used across neurodevelopmental and mental health services to understand and manage challenging behaviour, NbR is a system of behaviour support in and of itself. In fact, while NbR and PBS are both schools of behaviour support, with their origins rooted in learning theories and applied behaviour analysis, the model of NbR pre-dates the conception of modern PBS. Both systems share key similarities, as they both seek to maximise autonomy and skills development in their respective populations. However, the focus and application of NbR differs in a number of respects:

1 The needs of people with an acquired brain injury are typically different to those with neurodevelopmental disorders and NbR takes into consideration the neuropsychological profile and deficits of the individual in more detail.
2 NbR focuses on the re-learning of pro-social skills within an environment that is specifically designed to maximise therapeutic potential and minimise neurocognitive handicap.
3 NbR emphasises the role of neurocognitive factors in the maintenance of challenging behaviour, and learning theories play a key role in managing their influence through behavioural support planning.
4 NbR is rooted in principles of behaviourism and learning theory. PBS, while drawing on such principles, applies it to a lesser extent, and has greater emphasis on the improvement of quality of life, as well as the development of communication skills.
5 PBS primarily focuses on the management of behavioural antecedents, whereas NbR also considers behavioural consequences, with the understanding that challenging behaviour often serves an avoidance or escape function.
6 NbR considers the 'frontal lobe paradox' (Walsh, 1985) as a characteristic of ABI and, as such, NbR is better placed to manage this phenomenon than PBS. This phenomenon, sometimes referred to as the 'knowing-doing dissociation' (Teuber, 2009), refers to how some people with ABI may have significant difficulties in attending to everyday tasks such as cooking, taking medication, or self-care, but may show little by way of insight and may present in interviews (and assessments of capacity) as more able due to their unimpaired language skills.

Not all neurological services provide NbR as described in this chapter. However, while other neurological services tend to focus to a greater extent on a person's functional, psychological and emotional rehabilitation, they do often observe behavioural disturbance that requires intervention. The authors advocate for the use of the skills taught by NbR in these contexts given the evidence base that supports their use. However, in recent years there has been an attempt to adapt the broader PBS model for use with such a population.

The term PBS+PLUS has been used to describe the application of the PBS framework with people exhibiting challenging behaviour post-brain injury. However, at the time of writing, there have been comparatively few research studies that have aimed to validate this approach. Ponsford et al. (2022) compared a group of individuals with ABI receiving PBS+PLUS support with a group who were receiving minimal support and were on a treatment waiting list over a 12-month period. The authors concluded that they were unable to identify PBS+PLUS as being more effective than that received by the control group, as the latter exhibited similar improvements in behaviour. However, the key difference was in the confidence of close others in addressing challenging behaviour in the PBS+PLUS group. Other studies, such as that by Gould et al. (2021) have provided information on its use through qualitative review of case studies. As such, it remains too early to determine whether PBS+PLUS effectively reduces the frequency and intensity of challenging behaviour in the long term.

In view of the above, we consider NbR to be the most appropriate, evidence-based model on which to base a service whose primary aim is to manage challenging behaviour. However, services where this is not the primary aim can also learn much from elements of the approach.

Neurobehavioural support

Behaviour support in NbR services is reliant on a number of key elements to ensure successful outcomes, including: the provision of a structured environment filled with opportunities for learning; adherence to a transdisciplinary approach, where clinicians share responsibility for interventions, thereby creating a therapeutic culture; and the consistent application of behavioural reinforcements/contingencies by all staff involved in the individual's care. Each of these domains comes with its own challenges in application but should be underpinned by clear, concise behaviour support plans that prescribe how staff can deliver the required interventions.

There are three key concepts that should be considered in order to deliver effective neurobehavioural support.

Key concept 1: Assessment of challenging behaviour

An integral part of any behavioural support system is having a robust assessment of the person and their specific needs. This typically includes a battery of neuropsychological and psychometric measures. However, an assessment of the particular challenging behaviours in question should also be completed from the point of admission to any service, typically referred to as a 'functional behaviour assessment'. This seeks to determine the underlying functions of a particular behaviour, with the understanding that challenging behaviour is a means of communication of an underlying function, such as the desire to gain social attention, to gain tangible goods, to meet one's sensory needs, or to escape or avoid an aversive stimulus. It is only through a robust analysis of behavioural data that appropriate interventions can be designed to meet the needs of the person.

Functional behaviour assessment was developed as part of the discipline of applied behaviour analysis as a means of collecting information regarding the challenging behaviour, and its antecedents and consequences, as well as drawing conclusions as to the functions of a particular behaviour. Typically, such an assessment would also seek to collate information regarding the setting events, time, presence of others, frequency and intensity of challenging behaviours that can help clinicians to form an understanding about which interventions may mitigate risk and shape the person's behaviour.

The use of FBA has been well documented in the academic research. Arguably, the majority of research has been completed in the context of neurodevelopmental disorders. However, its use in ABI populations, and particularly in the context of NbR, has been described through many empirical studies that have evidenced its importance in obtaining good therapeutic outcomes. A starting point for such an assessment is the application of empirically validated behavioural observation measures that seek to record accurately a range of variables for further analysis. Tools such as the Overt Aggression Scale – Modified for Neurorehabilitation (Alderman, Knight and Morgan, 1997) and St Andrews Sexual Behaviour Assessment (Knight et al., 2008) have been designed specifically for use in ABI populations and NbR services, unlike many other measures used for FBA in other non-ABI populations. In addition, these tools benefit from a standardised approach with clear and succinct definitions of potential challenging behaviours that aid consistency in staff recordings. The OAS-MNR considers four types of challenging behaviour (verbal aggression, physical aggression against self, physical aggression against others, and damage to property) and four levels of potential intensity (from minor to serious), in addition to setting events, antecedents and interventions that have been used, whether successfully or unsuccessfully. Research has supported its inter-rater reliability in ABI populations (Alderman, 2003).

Key concept 2: Designing and implementing interventions

The behavioural data collected from the aforementioned observational measures support clinicians in developing clear hypotheses regarding the functions of the challenging behaviour, after which behavioural strategies can be considered that seek to shape behaviour and risk. Learning theories, primarily operant conditioning, procedural learning and errorless learning, are typically drawn upon to support decisions about interventions.

Operant learning, a core part of radical behaviourism (Skinner, 1953; Skinner, 1974), posits that learning occurs through experience of interaction with the physical and social world, with the likelihood of a repeated behaviour related to the pleasant or unpleasant consequence experienced. Operant learning methods have been cited by many studies as being effective in the management of neurobehavioural disability and plays a central role in the administration of NbR.

Once a hypothesis has been reached regarding the function of a challenging behaviour, a clearly defined goal should be determined that will help the person to establish better control over their behaviour in different situations. Operant learning methods, which can be employed by all members of the transdisciplinary team, are then advised; they should be recorded and communicated in a clear and concise manner.

Transdisciplinary teams can influence the trajectory of behaviour through operant learning methods by rewarding a behaviour (positive or negative reinforcement) or through extinction, where the expected reward is withheld (often referred to as 'Time Out on The Spot'). As such, the aim is to strengthen adaptive behaviours and skills, to downplay challenging behaviour (as far as risk allows), and to support the person in finding alternative means of having their needs met. The use of punishment strategies has also been documented in the research. However, given concerns about clinical ethics, the use of punishment as a means of learning (or re-learning) skills is no longer supported.

While the use of reinforcement techniques is central to the application of the operant model, those in NbR services also benefit from being provided with regular feedback throughout the day regarding their behaviour and progress. The transparency of such feedback aids not only learning, but also the development and maintenance of therapeutic relationships, without which reinforcements may lack power.

Clinicians should be mindful that, when using techniques such as extinction, there may be an 'extinction burst' which sees a temporary re-escalation of the challenging behaviour. This can often be a worrying time for the staff working with a given person, as they may be observing or, indeed, subject to, aggression or other forms of challenging behaviour. However, with continued application of the behavioural strategies, teams can expect a reduction in the frequency and severity of the behaviour. It is at this stage of treatment that staff require additional support in the form of reflective practice and supervision to ensure there is an understanding of the need to persevere.

Key concept 3: Behaviour support plans

In PBS, prescribed care plans outline the primary, secondary and tertiary interventions required to support an individual. These broadly translate to: (i) those interventions that aid improvement in quality of life and well-being; (ii) interventions that seek to mitigate the escalation of crises; and (iii) restrictive interventions that are designed to ensure the safety of the individual and others. However, in NbR, behaviour support takes a more focused and goal-centred approach. Any plans should be clear and concise in order to maximise their application; the provision of behaviour support plans that are of a significant length may have a detrimental effect on their application.

Neurobehavioural support plans should include information pertaining to the following.

Operational definition of the behaviour

In order to deliver effective interventions, it is important to have a clearly defined behaviour that the given team is aiming to shape. The operational definition should provide a clear and concise summary of the behaviour in question that all staff, and the person, can understand. Tools such as the OAS-MNR (Alderman, Knight and Morgan, 1997) offer predetermined operational definitions that can be used for this purpose.

Outcome of direct and/or indirect functional behaviour assessment

This provides a context for supporting staff by outlining the functions of the challenging behaviour and any other relevant findings from the functional behaviour assessment.

Clear explanation of the intervention(s) utilised

This section of a support plan should outline in clear terms how staff should look at both providing positive reinforcement for pro-social behaviours and responding to challenging behaviours (e.g., with the use of TOOTs). Where there is a special programme in place, the support plan should also outline the frequency of feedback to be provided, in addition to how it should be done, and by whom. Reference should be provided as to the method of recording of any challenging behaviours.

Evaluation of the intervention

A clear schedule for how clinicians will evaluate the efficacy of the interventions described should be provided. Any evaluation strategy should seek to regularly reflect on the trajectory of the behaviour, as well as how staff might be supported. It may also be important to highlight the need for any restrictive interventions, which should of course be seen as a last resort. Such restrictive interventions may include the use of segregation or restraint, taking into consideration the person's best interests, including any known physical health issues.

Withdrawal and generalisation

Interventions should be designed to be time-limited and goal-driven. As such, a neurobehavioural support plan should outline how the suggested intervention(s) will be withdrawn or minimised once the goal has been achieved.

Case example: David

David was a 25-year-old man, who sustained a TBI as a passenger in a road traffic collision (RTC) two years previously. Prior to his TBI, David had left education at 18 years of age and went on to work as an estate agent. Following his acute treatment for his TBI in a major trauma centre, he was referred back home to live with his partner. However, due to several incidents of physical aggression towards property and people within the community, he was admitted to a psychiatric unit. The service developed a PBS plan that outlined how staff could utilise positive reinforcement and extinction methods, but this met with minimal success. This is unsurprising as the literature finds that behaviour modification interventions using such approaches for aggression may be unsuccessful in cases of dysexecutive syndrome (see Alderman, Fry and Youngson, 1995).

As these interventions had not been successful, David was referred to a specialist neurorehabilitation unit. Neurocognitive testing revealed that his IQ was in the average range and in keeping with pre-morbid predictions on formal tests. However, he had specific cognitive vulnerabilities in aspects of executive functioning, namely attention, working memory, insight and self-monitoring, and he had difficulties regulating his emotions and behaviour. He also scored highly on a measure of depression. Functional assessment of his aggressive behaviour was completed using the Overt Aggression Scale – Modified for Neurorehabilitation, indicating that David would engage in verbal and physical aggression towards others, typically in response to the rehabilitation team inviting him to attend rehabilitation sessions. OAS-MNR data was shared with David and he expressed surprise at the frequency of incidents. It was formulated that the aggressive behaviour he was engaging in was secondary to the presence of dysexecutive syndrome and his adjustment to his TBI.

A behaviour support plan was formulated by the team, led by a consultant clinical neuropsychologist. This made reference to structured, timetabled rehabilitation sessions that included psychoeducation regarding TBI and psychotherapy to focus on psychosocial adjustment, and also to a positive reinforcement programme with social and tangible reinforcers to increase the likelihood of David attending sessions. In addition, a response-cost programme was noted in the behaviour support plan to target his aggression, and this was discussed with him and with his supporting staff. Response-cost has an evidence base in such cases and successfully circumvented David's specific cognitive needs. Monitoring on the OAS-MNR revealed that, over time, the severity and frequency of David's aggression reduced, with him enjoying and responding well to the positive reinforcement for engagement in his rehabilitation.

Challenges in the implementation of neurobehavioural support

The implementation of any effective therapeutic system, whether in inpatient or community services, is often filled with challenges, and behaviour support is no exception. Services should always be mindful of such issues and seek to mitigate any risks involved, as they can have a detrimental impact on a person's therapeutic pathway.

Client relationships and influence

Inpatient services that specialise in the treatment of people with neurobehavioural disability by definition comprise placements for multiple patients in the same ward or in the same building. Therapeutic programmes often seek to provide resocialisation, with the aim of providing social opportunities for patients that help them to build or regain not only social skills but also tolerance and impulse control. However, this can also pose challenges, as patients may struggle to relate to one another or to tolerate each other's behaviour or presence. It is this phenomenon that typically generates concerns around the safeguarding of individuals and that many neurorehabilitation services find difficult to manage (Alderman and Wood, 2013). As such, NbR services seek to ensure there are: (i) consideration of patient mix and behaviours prior to admission; (ii) clear care plans that provide structure and clear expectations; and (iii) staff training that builds staff knowledge and confidence in the application of restrictive practices should all other interventions be unsuccessful.

Family support

Neurobehavioural disability can have a significant impact on a person's relationships. As such, engaging families and carers is vital in the rehabilitation pathway for this population, especially as research suggest that challenging behaviour can persist for many years post-injury, and in some cases can even deteriorate further (Brooks et al., 1987; Kelly et al., 2008). Services should aim to include family members as part of the transdisciplinary team where feasible. Family members often have vital knowledge about the person's pre-morbid personality and behaviour and can also provide vital social support for the person post-discharge.

It is acknowledged, however, that family members may have struggled to cope previously with the stress caused by the person's challenging behaviour, which can pose a barrier to their involvement. While the authors acknowledge that not all services may have the facility to provide direct support for families, their continued positive mental health and empowerment to be involved in the patient's support network should be viewed as a key feature of the therapeutic programme, as patients with social support are more likely to have positive outcomes.

Staff training

NbR services should prioritise the regular, ongoing training of staff, particularly in terms of understanding ABI and NBD as well as behaviour support in this unique context. A focus on learning theory helps support staff to better understand the rationale for sometimes challenging interventions, which can help give consistency in application. Without this background knowledge, staff may reject neurobehavioural support plans due to a lack of appreciation of why they might be integral to the person's treatment. In addition, attendance at training events helps staff members to build confidence in their skill set and motivation to utilise approved techniques (e.g., Ashworth, Mooney and Tully, 2016).

Consistency of care

Consistency of care is often seen by clinicians as one of the most challenging of all potential barriers to effective treatment, regardless of the therapeutic model at play. However, ensuring that all staff receive robust ABI and behaviour support training, having effective and visible leadership on every shift and ensuring effective means of communication between shifts/teams can help to mitigate any drift in the application of interventions.

The use of competency frameworks or similar to help guide staff to understand their remit and skills required, which should be routinely monitored by senior registered clinicians, can support team members to establish a clear set of expectations about how to perform their roles in a given service.

However, the most commonly cited factor to impact adversely on consistency of care is that of communication, which can include the format and efficiency of handover meetings and opportunities for formal and informal discussions (or meetings specifically focusing on the client), including team formulations and care reviews. Ensuring such issues are considered and processes put in place to mitigate communication problems is vital in developing and maintaining an NbR service.

Transdisciplinary working

The transdisciplinary team is considered to be a central agent of behavioural change in NbR services. It is a form of collaborative working where traditional professional boundaries are more integrated and roles are shared with the patient in order to improve the delivery of the core therapeutic programme. Unidisciplinary approaches are arguably more prevalent in healthcare services, however, with only a few clinicians receiving exposure to the scientific skills and team processes necessary to collaborate successfully in teams of colleagues from widely disparate disciplines and fields (Hall et al., 2012). As such, those more familiar with a unidisciplinary approach may find it difficult to adapt to new ways of working without clear guidance and/or training.

Reflective practice and supervision

Clinical supervision is an important part of a clinician's working practice, with many of the professional regulatory bodies citing it to be a core requirement for registration. However, the provision of effective supervision for all staff, including those who are not subject to professional registrations, is key in the implementation and maintenance of a successful service. Neurobehavioural services should ensure that there are systems in place to provide regular supervision for all staff members, and to embed this into a shared culture of enquiry and support.

Similarly, the importance of reflective practice sessions for staff should not be underestimated. Reflective practice allows professionals to come together in order to share their collective knowledge and to aid teams in identifying complex clinical issues that will be the focus of interventions. In addition, such sessions are helpful in obtaining a helicopter view of staff well-being issues and to provide support and direction that may mitigate burnout.

Social climate

Social climate in the context of healthcare settings has been subject to many definitions over the years, with numerous methods of measurement referenced in the empirical literature. Research has also used the terms ward culture, atmosphere or therapeutic milieu, to describe the social interactions, relationships and impact of the physical environment on outcomes (Ekvall and Ryhammar, 1998; Nicholls et al., 2015). Research suggests that a positive social climate can result in better therapeutic outcomes in multiple populations including acute mental health (Dickens et al., 2022), forensic mental health (Doyle, Quayle and Newman, 2017), learning disability (Langdon, Budd and Swift, 2006; Willets, Mooney and Blagden, 2014) and older adults (McCann, Baird and Muir-Cochrane, 2015).

NbR seeks to promote a 'relentlessly positive' culture, where positive reinforcement of pro-social behaviours can flourish, and where staff and client well-being is maximised. As such, the concept of social climate, and how to develop a positive and proactive culture, are of the utmost importance. While there are many factors that influence the development of social climate and culture, arguably the provision of clear roles and guidance for staff, effective support and supervision and visible leadership are considered to be crucial.

Summary and practical implications

While NbR services typically offer interventions for a range of cognitive, emotional and functional problems, the provision of treatment that seeks to reduce the frequency and intensity of challenging behavioural support is the primary focus.

The concept of 'positive behaviour support', has become commonplace in mental health and neurodevelopmental services as a system to guide the application of interventions that enhance quality of life and teach new skills to a person. However, given the nature of most acquired brain injuries, behaviour support in the context of NbR services differs from that provided in other clinical services, with greater focus on learning theories, behavioural consequences and consideration of often complex cognitive factors. Indeed, the format of PBS typically used in neurodevelopmental services has, at the time of writing, received only limited validation in ABI populations, and so clinicians are encouraged to consider the unique focus provided by NbR services in achieving the goal of supporting challenging behaviour.

Services operating an NbR model and, indeed, any modern healthcare service can experience multiple challenges in the implementation of behaviour support approaches. Ensuring prescribed care plans have the appropriate content and that these are consistently applied are among the key challenges that require consideration and maintenance, as well as providing staff with specialist training and supervisory support. However, the ability to overcome such barriers and to operate the NbR model has been shown to provide good outcomes for those exhibiting challenging behaviour as a result of acquired brain injury.

References

Alderman, N. (2001). Management of challenging behaviour. In R.Ll. Wood and T. McMillan (eds), *Neurobehavioural Disability and Social Handicap Following Traumatic Brain Injury*. Hove: Psychology Press.

Alderman, N. (2003). Rehabilitation of behaviour disorders. In B.A. Wilson (ed.), *Neuropsychological Rehabilitation: Theory and Practice*. Lisse, The Netherlands: Swets and Zeitlinger.

Alderman, N., Fry, R. and Youngson, H.A. (1995). Improvement of self-monitoring skills, reduction of behaviour disturbance and the dysexecutive syndrome: Comparison of response cost and a new programme of self-monitoring training. *Neuropsychological Rehabilitation, 5* (3), 193–221.

Alderman, N., Knight, C. and Henman, C. (2002). Aggressive behaviour observed within a neurobehavioural rehabilitation service: Utility of the OAS-MNR in clinical audit and applied research. *Brain Injury, 16* (6), 469–489.

Alderman, N., Knight, C. and Morgan, C. (1997). Use of a modified Overt Aggression Scale in the measurement and assessment of aggressive behaviours following brain injury. *Brain Injury, 11* (7), 503–523.

Alderman, N. and Wood, R.Ll. (2013). Neurobehavioural approaches to the rehabilitation of challenging behaviour. *NeuroRehabilitation, 32*, 761–770.

Ashworth, S., Mooney, P. and Tully, R. (2016). Adapted DBT programme for individuals with intellectual disabilities and problems managing emotions: Staff awareness training. *Advances in Mental Health and Intellectual Disabilities, 10* (3), 185–198.

Brooks, D.N., McKinlay, W., Symington, C., Beattie, A. and Campsie, L. (1987). The effects of severe head injury upon patient and relative within seven years of injury. *Journal of Head Trauma Rehabilitation, 2*, 1–13.

Dickens, G.L., Johnson, A., Steel, K., Everett, B. and Tonkin, M. (2022). Interventions to improve social climate in acute mental health inpatient settings: Systematic review of content and outcomes. *SAGE Open Nursing, 8*. https://doi.org/10.1177/2377 9608221124291

Doyle, P., Quayle, E. and Newman, E. (2017). Social climate in forensic mental health settings: A systematic review of qualitative studies. *Aggression and Violent Behaviour, 36*, 118–136.

Dunlap, G. and Carr, E.G. (2007). Positive behavior support and developmental disabilities: A summary and analysis of research. In S.L. Odom, R.H. Horner, M.E. Snell and J. Blacher (eds), *Handbook of Developmental Disabilities*. New York: The Guilford Press.

Dunlap, G., Sailor, W., Horner, R.H. and Sugai, G. (2009). Overview and history of positive behaviour support. In W. Sailor, G. Dunlop, G. Sugai and R. Horner (eds), *Handbook of Positive Behaviour Support*. New York: Springer Publishing Company.

Ekvall, G.A. and Ryhammar, L. (1998). Leadership style, social climate and organizational outcomes: A study of a Swedish university college. *Creativity and Innovation Management, 7*, 126–130.

Gould, K.R., Ponsford, J.L., Hicks, A.J., Hopwood, M., Renison, B. and Feeney, T.J. (2021). Positive behaviour support for challenging behaviour after acquired brain injury: An introduction to PBS+PLUS and three case studies. *Neuropsychological Rehabilitation, 31* (1), 57–59.

Hall, K.L., Vogel, A.L., Stipelman, B.A., Stokols, D., Morgan, G. and Gehlert, S. (2012). A four-phase model of transdisciplinary team-based research: Goals, team processes, and strategies. *Translational Behavioral Medicine, 2* (4), 415–430.

Kelly, G., Brown, S., Todd, J. and Kremer, P. (2008). Challenging behaviour profiles of people with acquired brain injury living in community settings. *Brain Injury, 22* (6), 457–470.

Knight, C., Alderman, N., Johnson, C., Green, S., Birkett-Swan, L. and Yorston, G. (2008). The St Andrew's Sexual Behaviour assessment (SASBA): Development of a standardised recording instrument for the measurement and assessment of challenging sexual behaviour in people with progressive and acquired neurological impairment. *Neuropsychological Rehabilitation, 18*, 129–159.

Koegel, L.K., Koegel, R.Ll. and Dunlap, G. (eds) (1996). *Positive behavioral support: Including people with difficult behavior in the community*. Baltimore, MD: Paul H. Brookes Publishing Co.

Langdon, P.E., Budd, R. and Swift, A.L. (2006). Social climate within secure inpatient services for people with intellectual disabilities. *Journal of Intellectual Disability Research, 50* (11), 828–836.

Larkin, K.Y. and Zvolensky, M.J. (2001). Behaviour therapy. In M. Hersen and V.B. van Hasselt (eds), *Advanced Abnormal Psychology*. New York: Plenum Press.

McCann, T., Baird, J. and Muir-Cochrane, E.C. (2015). Social climate of acute old age psychiatry inpatient units: Staff perceptions within the context of patient aggression. *Journal of Psychiatric and Mental Health Nursing, 22* (2), 102–108.

Morgan, A.B. and Lilienfeld, S.O. (2000). A meta-analytic review of the relation between antisocial behaviour and neuropsychological measures of executive function. *Clinical Psychology Review, 20* (1), 113–156.

Nicholls, D., Kidd, K., Threader, J. and Hungerford, C. (2015). The value of purpose-built mental health facilities: Use of the ward atmosphere scale to gauge the link between milieu and physical environment. *International Journal of Mental Health Nursing, 24* (4), 286–294.

Ponsford, J.L., Hicks, A.J., Gould, K.R., Downing, M.G., Hopwood, M. and Feeney, T.J. (2022). Positive behaviour support for adults with acquired brain injury and challenging behaviour: A randomised controlled trial. *Annals of Physical and Rehabilitation Medicine, 65* (2), 101604.

Rao, V., Rosenberg, P., Bertrand, M., Salehinia, S., Spiro, J., Vaishani, S., Rastogi, P., Noll, K., Schretlen, D.J., Brandt, J., Cornwell, E., Makley, M. and Miles, Q.S. (2009).

Aggression after traumatic brain injury: Prevalence and correlates. *Journal of Neuropsychiatry and Clinical Neuroscience, 21* (4), 420–429.

Siever, L. (2008). Neurobiology of aggression and violence. *American Journal of Psychiatry, 165* (4), 429–442.

Skinner, B.F. (1953). *Science and Human Behaviour*. New York: Macmillan.

Skinner, B.F. (1974). *About Behaviourism*. New York: Vintage Books.

Teuber, H.L. (2009). The riddle of frontal lobe function in man. *Neuropsychology Review, 19* (1), 25–46.

Tonkonogy, J.M. (1991). Violence and temporal love lesion: Head CT and MRI data. *Journal of Neuropsychiatry and Clinical Neuroscience, 3* (2), 189–196.

Visscher, A.J.M., van Meijel, B., Stolker, J.J. and Nijman, H. (2011). Aggressive behaviour of inpatients with acquired brain injury. *Journal of Clinical Nursing, 20* (23–24), 3414–3422.

Walsh, K.W. (1985). *Understanding Brain Damage: A Primer of Neuropsychological Evaluation*. London: Longman Group.

Willets, L., Mooney, P. and Blagden, N. (2014). Social climate in learning disability services. *Journal of Intellectual Disabilities and Offending Behaviour, 5* (1), 24–37.

Williams, C., Wood, R.Ll., Alderman, N. and Worthington, A. (2020). The psychosocial impact of neurobehavioral disability. *Frontiers in Neurology, 11*, 119.

8 Management of aggression after acquired brain injury

Nick Alderman

Introduction

Aggression is arguably the most debilitating feature of neurobehavioural disability (see Chapter 1) (Fleminger, Greenwood and Oliver, 2006), which has a catastrophic impact on survivors, families and communities. It is negatively associated with functional abilities, care needs and participation in life roles, and it is is a frequently reported concern of family members underpinning social isolation, concern for the future and care-giver stress (Tam et al., 2015). Associations between aggression and offending after TBI have been reported in large scale population studies. Fazel et al. (2011) demonstrated violent crime was over-represented among people with TBI compared to the general population (8.8 vs 2.3 per cent), and in prison populations (Williams et al., 2010).

Aggression in rehabilitation services compromises the safety of others, increases vulnerability of the aggressor, and decreases the likelihood that full rehabilitation potential will be achieved. It explains why many clinicians dislike working with this group, and the risk of aggression often leads to exclusion from rehabilitation. When this happens, individuals gravitate to placements for management purposes as diverse as prison, forensic and secure mental health services, and nursing homes, ill-equipped to meet their needs (Alderman, 2017).

How much of a problem is it?

Studies investigating prevalence have variable results. For example, Tateno, Jage and Robinson (2003) found incidence varied between studies from as little as 11 per cent to as much as 96 per cent. This was attributed to lack of agreement on a standard definition of aggression. Other factors contributing to variability include the non-homogeneous nature of ABI and a range of methodological issues regarding how, when and in what context behaviour is measured.

For example, symptoms of NBD, including aggression, can increase over time (see Chapter 1), so the comparatively low frequency reported in studies conducted within months of injury is not a good predictor of later prevalence. Another confounding variable is misattributing the presence of undesirable behaviour as being a product of ABI, without understanding the base rate of

DOI: 10.4324/9781003083290-11

this in the neurologically healthy population. One study found prevalence of aggression amongst people with TBI and controls was surprisingly similar: 58 per cent of neurologically healthy people self-reported aggression that met the study criteria in comparison to 57 per cent of TBI survivors 60 months after injury. However, whilst overall rates were compatible, there were some key differences, most notably physical aggression was higher within the TBI group, including physical assaults on other people (19 per cent vs 4 per cent) (Baguley, Cooper and Felmingham, 2006). These data do support the hypothesis that behaviour change occurs as a consequence of ABI.

Context can also be a confounding factor; aggression varies in response to a range of variables, including situation and expectations. For example, Gould et al. (2019) found differences in aggressive behaviour among TBI survivors living at home and those in residential accommodation. Verbal and physical aggression were evident in both contexts. However, the range and severity of aggressive behaviour was greatest in residential settings. Aggression at home was associated with failures in social cognition, whereas in residential settings it was a response to, for example, prompting to perform personal care tasks. Aggression is also characteristic of people referred to specialist services for behaviour management purposes. Kelly et al. (2008) determined the type and severity of challenging behaviours in a cohort of ABI survivors referred to a community behaviour management service. Verbal aggression was most frequent (86 per cent of the sample); other forms of aggressive behaviour included aggression against people (41 per cent) and objects (35 per cent). As the time since injury was lengthy (mean 10 years, maximum 41 years), Kelly and colleagues concluded aggression is a long-term consequence of ABI.

A further example of how prevalence differs depending on context is evident through assessment of aggressive behaviour using the St Andrew's–Swansea Neurobehavioural Outcomes Scale (see Chapter 5; Alderman, Wood and Williams, 2011). In their study of 87 TBI survivors living in the community, Alderman, Williams and Wood (2021) found 40 per cent engaged in aggressive behaviour in the previous two-week period, beyond the threshold for neurologically healthy controls. In contrast, these researchers had previously reported all 100 participants in a neurobehavioural rehabilitation programme had met these criteria (Alderman, Wood and Williams, 2011). The finding that a significant minority of people with TBI were assessed as displaying more aggression than expected compared to healthy controls reflects a methodological strength of the SASNOS. Normative data regarding the presence of NBD-type symptoms were available as control subjects were also assessed on this measure. From these data, thresholds are available, so scores falling below these are known to be atypical of the general population.

Whilst prevalence is varied, when aggression is present it constitutes a chronic problem imposing a serious handicap and poor psychosocial outcome. Families find it especially distressing, and it is acknowledged as posing the greatest impediment to community integration in TBI survivors, even greater than the physical disabilities (Kelly et al., 2008).

What causes aggression after ABI?

Drivers of NBD were described in Chapter 1, having origins in neurological damage and neurocognitive impairment, further modified through interaction with various factors, including learning. Four principal explanations underpin post-ABI aggression.

1   Lesions to the prefrontal cortex and its connections with other brain structures are strongly associated with aggression. The orbito-temporal-limbic feedback loop is particularly implicated, with the inhibitory function of the cortex over the amygdala being disrupted, depriving the cognitive functions of their ability to suppress instinctive emotional reactions (Starkstein and Robinson, 1991). Aggressive behaviour is provoked by clear antecedents, resulting in a response that escalates quickly (Medd and Tate, 2000). Reduction in inhibitory control probably accounts for increased aggression in people with a pre-morbid history of violence (Dyer et al., 2006).

2   A further category of neurologically mediated aggression is the episodic dyscontrol syndrome (EDS), one of the post-traumatic temporo-limbic disorders. EDS aggression tends to be brief, 'out of character', and often without obvious triggers. If there is a trigger, it is usually minor and the magnitude of the behavioural response grossly out of proportion. Whilst those with EDS often express regret over their behaviour, the unexpected nature of the outburst has an adverse emotional impact upon families (Wood, 2001). Its development parallels post-traumatic epilepsy in that onset is marked by a delay (sometimes years) after injury and it shows little improvement over time. Anticonvulsant medication has a key role to play in management, which is discussed elsewhere (see Eames, 2001).

3   Neurocognitive impairment, especially executive function disorders, results in reduced ability to initiate the use of preserved abilities, monitor performance, and utilise feedback effectively to regulate behaviour. This generates a lack of 'error awareness' and consequently problems with social cognition. Social performance is characterised by disinhibition, impulsiveness, poor response to cues, and embarrassing 'odd' behaviour. Social failure results in increased frustration, loss of temper and aggression when there are difficulties with response inhibition, as described above (Alderman, 2003a).

4   Post-injury learning is highly important in the evolution of aggressive behaviour. Alderman (2007) showed how interactions between different patterns of neurocognitive impairment with various environmental factors resulted in dissociable types of aggression requiring different management approaches, whilst Rahman, Oliver and Alderman (2010) demonstrated how learning influences post-ABI results in aggression mainly serving either an avoidance/escape or attention-motivated function.

Chapter 1 also showed that principal drivers of behaviour are not limited to one factor, but invariably interact, and that behaviour is further shaped by additional variables. For example, neurologically mediated impulsive aggression is an outcome of TBI, particularly that resulting from rapid deceleration forces, where damage to prefrontal structures is especially vulnerable (as in (1) above). Probability of aggressive behaviour is increased when social cognition errors result from neurocognitive impairment (3) or as a consequence of post-injury learning (4). Regarding the last point, Chapter 2 showed how challenging behaviour is maintained through operant learning in the evolution of avoidance/escape and attention-motivated behaviours. Another important contributing factor is lack of meaningful routine and activity. Alderman (2007) found that physical assaults on other people most frequently took place when patients were not engaged in structured activity; furthermore, this aggression was most characterised by having no directly observable cause, being more severe, and requiring more restrictive interventions to manage it in comparison to that observed during structured activities.

How can post-ABI aggression be managed?

Interventions derived from learning theory are effective in the management of post-ABI challenging behaviour, including aggression (Ylvisaker et al., 2007; Wood and Alderman, 2011; Alderman, 2015). It provides a conceptual framework that facilitates a formulation-led approach to understanding relationships between behaviour with environmental contingencies and neurocognitive impairment. It will be recalled from Chapter 6 that drawing from the range of evidence-based techniques derived from new learning theory at the clinician's disposal, there are three broad approaches: those based on changing antecedent conditions; those based on changing responses to behaviour; and those based on increasing self-regulation through modifying internal cognitive mechanisms. It will further be recalled from Chapter 2 that the complexities underlying post-ABI behaviour change invariably necessitate incorporating approaches from two or more of the methods described in Chapter 6 in the form of multi-component interventions.

Application of the process model described in Chapter 2 enables assessment, formulation and construction of a behaviour support plan to manage aggression. However, because this behaviour arguably carries most risk, a conservative approach needs to be taken in deciding if the plan can be safely undertaken. Families and care staff may not have the necessary skills or confidence to take this on. Special caution must be taken when withholding a reinforcer that maintains aggression, as this is likely to result in an extinction burst characterised by an escalation in behaviour. It is strongly advised that, when there is risk of physical assaults on others, referral is made to NbR services; these have the capacity to safely manage extremes of behaviour.

Management of severe aggression – neurobehavioural rehabilitation

NbR was conceptualised over four decades ago to meet the needs of people with ABI whose challenging behaviour prevented engagement in neurorehabilitation. NbR creates conditions under which learning can take place and provides social opportunities where skills can be practised. Many challenging behaviours symptomatic of NBD, including aggression, are acquired post-injury to fulfil functions that are 'anti-rehabilitation', most notably those that are avoidance/escape or attention-motivated (Rahman, Oliver and Alderman, 2010). Early practitioners developed a framework for social interaction conceptualised to influence positively the diminished awareness of social rules arising from a reduced ability to self-regulate behaviour, typical from damage to the prefrontal cortex. Operant interventions reward desirable behaviours, providing a source of motivation and sense of achievement from engaging in therapeutic activities, and a source of systematic feedback to raise awareness when this is otherwise undermined by neurocognitive impairment (Wood, Alderman and Worthington, 2020).

Principal characteristics of NbR are as follows.

1 Expert knowledge regarding ABI and its outcomes.
2 Clinicians who are specialists in the application of methods derived from new learning theory and knowledge regarding constraints on this imposed by neurocognitive impairment.
3 A structured programme of meaningful activity and routine, offering patients the ability to practise skills taught in sessions in the context of normal social behaviour.
4 Availability of frequent feedback about behaviour and performance, that helps learning and promotes awareness and understanding of social handicap.
5 The ability to admit people under an appropriate legal framework (e.g., in England and Wales, most NbR services are registered as hospitals that have legal authority to detain and treat patients under the Mental Health Act (1983)).
6 A physical environment able to withstand severe challenging behaviour.
7 A clinical team trained in the use of physical intervention techniques and who understand the legal framework governing this.
8 A clinical team organised as a transdisciplinary team that maximises the effectiveness of all disciplines and the consistency with which interventions are delivered.
9 The provision of a 'relentlessly positive' social milieu promoting motivation, success and the context in which the least intrusive behaviour support plans are employed.
10 The integration of appropriate outcome and measurement instruments, within the clinical fabric of a service, that help identify goals, track progress and determine effectiveness.

A transdisciplinary team approach to rehabilitation

It is highly recommended that clinical teams providing any form of neurorehabilitation aspire to do so as a TDT. In NbR services, this provides a vehicle through which all team members consistently apply behaviour support plans and rehabilitation programmes. It is ideally suited for optimising service delivery to the complex needs of people with ABI who require therapeutic input beyond that of a single discipline. For example, whilst the primary goal may fall under the domain of the physiotherapist, difficulties with communication and behaviour require concurrent input from speech and language therapy and psychology, with the result that a plan is created by all three disciplines working closely together. Because learning is more successful when plans are implemented whenever required, other team members are trained to implement it, including nurses and carers. This has two important advantages. First, frequent implementation of the plan whenever it is needed helps ensure learning occurs as quickly as possible until the new behaviour or skill becomes engrained as a habit. Second, because the plan is consistently used whenever and wherever needed, generalisation across settings is more likely.

A TDT shares roles across disciplinary boundaries, so that communication, interaction and cooperation are maximised among team members. It is characterised by commitment to teach, learn and work together to implement coordinated services. This leads to a mutual vision or 'shared meaning' within the team and results in: (i) shared assessment and goal selection; (ii) close cooperation and exchange of information, knowledge and skills across the entire team; and (iii) 'role release', characterised by intervention strategies traditionally delivered by specific disciplines, being implemented by the entire team under the supervision of team members whose disciplines are normally accountable for those practices (King, Strachan, Tucker, Duwyn, Desserud, and Shillington, 2009). The approach fosters consistency, pursuit of meaningful patient-centred functional goals, and delivery of rehabilitation 24 hours a day, seven days a week.

The characteristics of NbR enable the creation of enriched, person-centred social environments within which behaviour support plans are consistently applied and positive social climates promote therapeutic relationships associated with good treatment outcomes (Alderman and Groucott, 2012). The provision of behavioural interventions in this way is antagonistic to aggression while actively promoting new learning, skill acquisition, independence and a collaborative approach to rehabilitation, giving patients more choice, control and freedom as they progress. Alderman and Knight (2017) demonstrated how exposure to a positive social climate, underpinned by operant behaviour management interventions, impacts on aggression. They used the Overt Aggression Scale – Modified for Neurobehavioural Rehabilitation (Alderman, Knight and Morgan, 1997) (see Chapter 5) to demonstrate a reduction in aggressive behaviour of 50 patients admitted to one of three NbR services; at discharge, there was a 90 per cent reduction. Alderman (2015) described the reduction in aggression in three separate cases. Aggressive behaviour was tracked using the OAS-MNR alongside a quantitative indicator of rehabilitation expectations. All cases demonstrated a reduction in aggression while increasing rehabilitation expectations.

Creating environments that support behaviour change

The characteristics of NbR create person-centred, positive environments. They support new learning through systems that circumvent neurocognitive barriers through structure, routine and regular feedback. Taking steps that emulate, as far as possible, these characteristics in other neurological services provides a context that supports behaviour support plans. Practical steps to pursue this include the following.

1   *Changing antecedent conditions*: specifically, implementing a programme of meaningful activity, including social opportunities, encouraging the team to engage positively whenever possible with patients, and being consistent with regard to expectations about what patients can and cannot do for themselves.
2   *Changing responses to behaviour*: namely, giving patients positive feedback about what they do well together with unconditional feedback regarding aggressive behaviour, social reinforcement following any behaviours commensurate with rehabilitation and community living, and avoiding social reinforcement of aggressive behaviour.

Making it happen – from plan to implementation

A behaviour support plan is the crowning achievement of the initial stages of the process model. However, the success of the very best intervention is dependent on the ability of others to deliver it as intended. Anxieties about trying to change aggressive behaviour will undoubtedly exist and these must be addressed before the plan begins. The team should be encouraged to embark on treatment in the spirit of a collaborative venture, in which everybody feels able to contribute ideas and share concerns. Progress should be regularly reviewed, and members should be encouraged to view the plan as everybody's domain – perception of group ownership embraces the expectation that all have responsibility to implement the plan when required.

In addition to aspiring to team ownership, Alderman (2001) suggested the effective delivery of programmes was further dependent on what were described as 'the three Cs':

1   *Consistency*. For new learning to occur it is essential that all team members consistently implement the intervention as the standard response to aggression. Deviation risks exacerbating behaviour.
2   *Clarity*. Knowing when to intervene underlines why behaviour is specified in operational terms. Using definitions of behaviour provided by the OAS-MNR is especially helpful (e.g., 'the following procedure will be used immediately following any verbal aggression VA3 and VA4'). Similarly, the procedure to follow must be clearly and succinctly described so that everybody follows it consistently.

3   *Contingencies.* What happens immediately in response to aggression is critical. This is the 'business end' of the behaviour support plan. All behaviour results in consequences that encourage it through reinforcement, or discourage it by withholding a reinforcer, punishing it, or result in nothing changing (see Chapter 2). The intervention defines exactly what the contingencies to aggressive behaviour are – most commonly, provision of verbal prompts, provision of a tangible item, removing a tangible item, and ignoring behaviour.

In addition to training, a document that accompanies the patient throughout the period the plan is in operation will contain information to inform team members of 'the three Cs'. This should be restricted to the information needed to enable the plan to be operated. All other information, such as detailed assessment measures, should be stored in the clinical record. The plan should not exceed one side of A4 paper. The intervention should be concisely described, typically comprising the operational definition of the behaviour, the goal of the plan, what to do when the behaviour is observed, who delivers the required contingencies, and how it is recorded. See Alderman (2001) for an example of this. All team members will receive training; regular refresher sessions help maintain consistency and the ethos of shared ownership. Changes to the plan are always communicated to the whole team to ensure compliance and consistency are maintained.

Differential reinforcement is useful

When assessment indicates aggression serves a specific function, use of the variants of differential reinforcement discussed in Chapter 6 have special relevance, and are frequently employed in managing avoidance/escape and attention-motivated behaviours (Wood and Alderman, 2011). Differential reinforcement of incompatible behaviour rewards behaviour incompatible with aggression – for example, through use of a fixed interval reinforcement schedule, when reward is available at the end of a specific time-period providing no aggressive behaviour has been observed.

Differential reinforcement of other behaviour is useful when frequency of aggression is too high to reward its absence practically during a designated time-period. Instead, reward is contingent on some other behaviour occurring, regardless of whether aggression is observed. This is helpful when a plan is initially implemented in order to create conditions of success that would not be possible when aggression is continuous. Concurrent reduction in aggression that parallels reinforcement of other behaviour often occurs, and subsequently enables later use of DRI.

Differential reinforcement of low rates of behaviour provides an alternative to DRO by setting a target frequency of aggression for a period of time; a count is maintained and if, at the end of a time-period, the number counted is less than the target, reinforcement is administered. It is good practice to ensure the initial target is achievable with no or little effort being exerted by the patient; this sets conditions for success and encourages their 'buy in' from the start. When the target is achieved, it is increased for the next session at a rate the patient can achieve, until ideally aggression is no longer evident. The load on a patient's memory is reduced by giving feedback about progress at short, fixed intervals.

Examples of the management of aggressive behaviour

The rest of this chapter will be concerned with practical recommendations regarding the management of aggression that fulfils two frequent functions post-ABI, avoidance/escape and attention-motivated behaviour (Rahman, Oliver and Alderman, 2010). The methods are drawn from operant learning theory; whilst they have an evidence base for management of post-ABI challenging behaviour and are therefore not exclusively concerned with the reduction of aggression, they have been found to be especially relevant for this purpose.

Managing avoidance/escape and attention-motivated aggressive behaviour

When assessment associates a function with a behaviour, a bespoke behaviour support plan is required. In Chapter 2, Table 2.1 summarises the contingencies operating to sustain the two most frequent categories of function-driven aggressive behaviour: avoidance-escape motivated aggression, maintained by negative reinforcement (patient behaviour) and positive punishment (carer behaviour); and attention-motivated aggression through positive reinforcement (patient) and negative reinforcement (carer). Behaviour support plans reduce aggression by disrupting these contingencies and changing the behaviour of both patients and carers. Where aggression fulfils an avoidance/escape function, behaviour is negatively reinforced for as long as it succeeds in reducing demands made by clinicians and carers, so these expectations must be maintained. When aggression is positively reinforced by attention from others, this must be withheld.

Multi-component interventions to manage aggression maintaining either of these functions typically draw from the following.

Changing antecedent conditions

1 To increase consistency, especially in inexperienced teams, the behaviour support plan is implemented by a small group, whose members are motivated to take the programme on, perhaps as a 'trial' to demonstrate efficacy. Limiting this to a specific session or task until its efficacy is known helps encourage wider uptake of the plan.

2 Avoidance/escape behaviour is often task-focused – for example, participating in sessions or completing personal activities of daily living. Varying expectations regarding what the person can do independently and how much assistance they need contributes to inconsistency, resulting in

intermittent reinforcement of aggression. This is improved by standardising expectations by breaking a task down into constituent parts to form a sequence of steps that staff can follow. Verbally prompting the patient through each task-part also has the advantage of incorporating errorless learning, further assisting learning.

3 Patients often associate anxieties or historical negative experiences with particular disciplines. Being asked to 'attend physiotherapy', for example, may constitute a setting event that increases the likelihood of aggression. This can be reduced by labelling areas associated with disciplines neutrally and aligning the timetable to these descriptors. For example, using colours such as 'red room' and 'green room', as opposed to physiotherapy and psychology.

4 Disguising therapy within functional and recreational activities reduces avoidance/escape-motivated behaviour associated with disciplines. A group session in which patients and carers play a board game can be a vehicle for addressing multiple rehabilitation goals such as good posture, social communication and reinforcing desirable behaviours, in which carers act as positive role models.

5 When a patient is aggressive as a response to a request to attend a therapy session, this can be held in the space they are already in, such as a day room, lounge or bedroom. Graded exposure to higher expectations in subsequent sessions, for example by increasing session time in 5-minute increments, weakens the function of aggressive behaviour, especially if patients learn to associate these activities with pleasant outcomes.

Changing responses to behaviour

1 Social praise is frequently used to reinforce behaviours incompatible with aggression. Care is needed to deliver praise in a way a patient does not perceive as patronising or unwelcome. Social praise contributes to re-learning associations between behaviour and social rules governing behaviour.

2 Unless the behaviour support plan prescribes a different response, carers need to be consistent in maintaining expectations while (as far as possible) making no response to aggression using TOOTS. As soon as aggressive behaviour stops, carers should re-engage with the patient and social reinforcement should be made available again.

3 The inclusion of a procedure using tangible and social reinforcement to incentivise desirable behaviour is a potentially important component of the plan, especially when social reinforcement and TOOTS prove ineffective. Using one of the differential reinforcement variants described earlier can be especially effective. DRL is employed in management of avoidance/escape (Alderman and Knight, 1997) and attention-motivated aggression (Watson et al., 2001) by reinforcing successively lower rates of aggressive behaviour. When a task-part sequence is employed to prompt a patient through the steps to complete a functional activity associated with aggression, DRO can be used to reinforce cooperation with following prompts; aggression is

ignored and does not contribute to whether reinforcement is earned. Alderman, Shepherd and Youngson (1992) successfully employed DRO in this way to reinforce the completion of tasks in physiotherapy that were previously associated with increased anxiety and aggressive behaviour, resulting in escape. DRI is subsequently used to reinforce the complete absence of aggression.

Increasing self-regulation

1 A verbal script assists the development of self-regulation and improved inhibitory control. For example, when using a task-part sequence checklist to learn a skill, a carer verbally prompts a patient to complete a functional task by reading each of these aloud, working through the sequence. The patient is prompted to repeat the task-part before carrying out the action, improving self-regulation, enhancing learning and reducing anxiety previously associated with the task (see Alderman, 2015).
2 Self-regulation is improved by modifying cognitive schemata associated with aggression. For example, Burgess and Alderman (1990) described the case of SJ whose anticipatory anxiety before washing and dressing resulted in verbal aggression and physical aggression against himself (beating his chest with his fist). As part of a multi-component intervention, SJ was frequently prompted during the task to repeat a written phrase presented on a card. Repetition assisted in modifying the dysfunctional cognitive schemata associated with anxiety and aggression with an alternative belief, elicited from SJ by using a simplified form of cognitive restructuring. Increased self-control resulted in significant reduction of anxiety and aggressive behaviour, which continued after the intervention was withdrawn.

Case examples

Two cases will be described to illustrate how various combinations of these methods can be combined successfully to create a behaviour support plan for the management of avoidance/escape and attention-motivated behaviour. These cases were resident in care home settings.

Escape/avoidance motivated aggression: NR

NR (Alderman, 2003b) sustained a severe TBI, characterised one year post-injury by severe cognitive and physical impairments, and was heavily dependent on carers. Expert opinion was that he had considerable rehabilitation potential but challenging behaviour prevented this. Verbal aggression and shouting were especially evident. Frustration-tolerance was low. Behaviour assessment revealed carers lacked consistency in managing NR. In physical tasks, expectations varied considerably regarding what he was expected to do independently. Response to verbal aggression varied. Functional analysis indicated that, when

NR was asked to complete a task independently, he was verbally aggressive and, as a consequence, most staff completed tasks for him. Consequently, the formulation concluded that verbal aggression served an avoidance/escape function.

A multi-component behaviour support plan drew from all three categories of intervention. *Changes to antecedent conditions*: (i) carers lacked experience in managing challenging behaviour, so a small group of volunteers took this on to maximise commitment and consistency; (ii) the intervention was limited to washing and dressing, to trial the programme and increase consistency; and carers' expectations were standardised by breaking the task down into 32 task-parts, each of which indicated when assistance was required. *Changing responses to behaviour*: (i) prodigious social praise for appropriate behaviour; (ii) downplaying verbal aggression using TOOTS and maintaining programme demands; (iii) a DRL intervention, targeting successively lower rates of verbal aggression to achieve an agreed reinforcer – a three-week assessment period found NR was verbally aggressive an average of 214 times, the initial target set was 300; (iv) feedback given at five-minute intervals regarding progress. Finally, *increasing self-regulation*: prior to completing each task-part, a carer read that step aloud and NR was asked to repeat this.

Results are shown in Figure 8.1. After 80 sessions, verbal aggression had fallen to a mean of 5.42, by which time NR had achieved greater independence in washing and dressing. Periodic follow-up, up to three years later, demonstrated the maintenance of these gains. Following this success, it was possible to ensure conditions of consistency that enabled this intervention to run throughout the whole day, with OAS-MNR recordings confirming a reduction

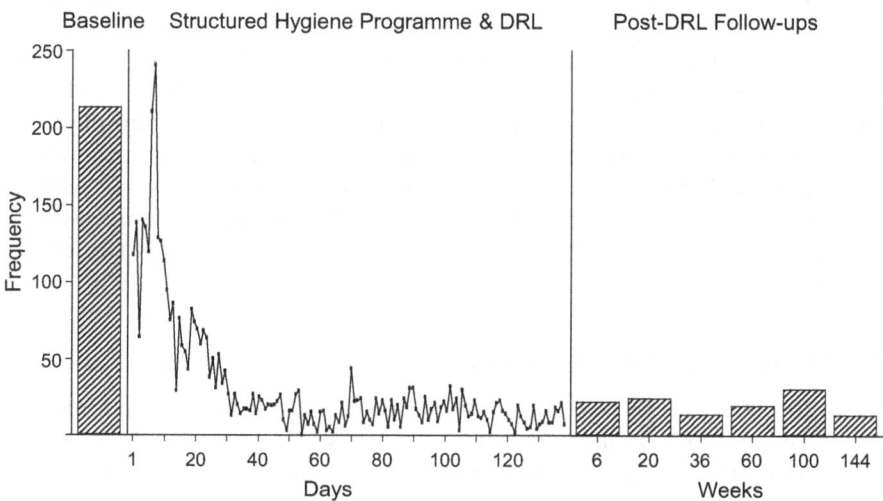

Figure 8.1 NR: reduction in OAS-MNR recordings while washing and dressing using a task-part sequence checklist and DRL.

in aggressive behaviour and full engagement with rehabilitation activities previously avoided. Increased autonomy and behaviour improvements enabled successful discharge to a community placement.

Attention-motivated behaviour: JH

JH (Watson et al., 2001) sustained a severe penetrating brain injury and multiple disabilities, including severe cognitive impairment and challenging behaviour. Physical aggression necessitated admission to an NbR service; after three years JH made sufficient improvement to be transferred to a residential setting to continue rehabilitation. Here, verbal aggression and occasional physical aggression were evident, characterised by shouting, swearing and threatening residents and carers. Behaviour was intimidating to the point that JH was avoided. Carers complained about working with him; and JH spent most of the day alone. Functional analysis confirmed aggression mostly lacked overt antecedents, and typically led to rebuke from carers. Acceptable requests to engage with other people were mostly ignored and JH remained socially isolated. The formulation concluded aggression principally served an attention-motivated function.

The multi-component intervention was as follows. *Changes to antecedent conditions*: included provision of meaningful activity through introduction of a programme of enjoyable activities, which extended to include rehabilitation sessions. *Changing responses to behaviour*: (i) encouragement of carers to interact positively with JH and respond to all requests that excluded verbal aggression; (ii) consistent use of TOOTS in response to aggression; (iii) provision of a DRL programme targeting successively lower rates of aggressive behaviour – the day was divided into four (subsequently five) time-periods and if JH's aggression did not exceed the target he earned a star, the number of stars accumulated were exchanged for tangible reinforcers he chose in the evening.

Figure 8.2 confirms the success of this plan, and it indicates key points at which expectations and changes in medication were made because of the decrease in aggression, including participation in group sessions and physical therapy. This also reflects that learning was slow, because of neurocognitive impairment, underlining the need for a consistent approach. After 85 weeks, JH successfully transferred to a house in the grounds of the care home, where, with the support of a care team, he successfully cohabited with two other residents.

Managing severe neurocognitive impairment

Finally, the issue of severe neurocognitive impairment will be briefly addressed. Aggressive behaviour occurring in the context of severe impairments in executive function, attentional controls and memory are more resistant to intervention. Time-out approaches, including TOOTS, may be ineffective because patients are unaware they are being ignored. Use of sophisticated interventions based on differential reinforcement fail because patients are unable to recall or

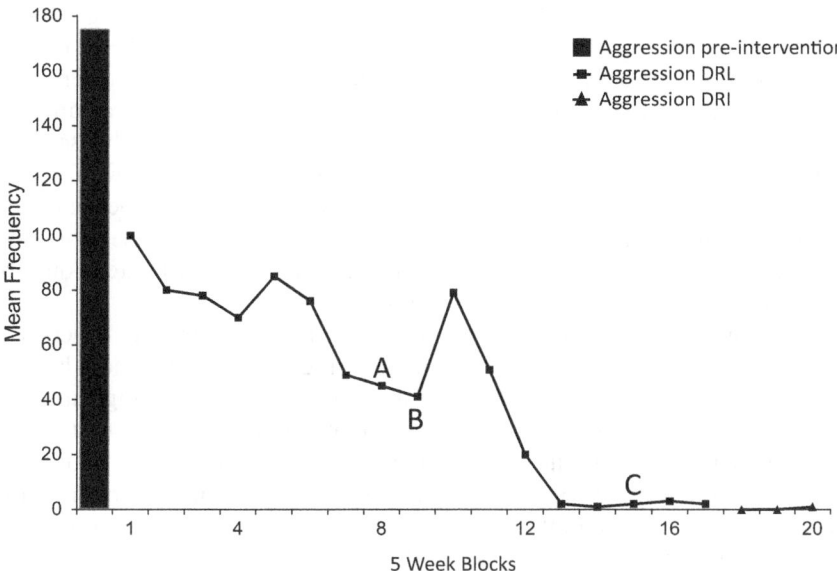

Figure 8.2 JH: reduction in OAS-MNR recordings using differential reinforcement. Key: A: time periods during day increased from 4 to 5, rehabilitation expectations increased; B: reduction in medication; C: transferred to house.

comprehend conditions leading to reinforcement, and they lack awareness when they are aggressive. Alderman and Burgess (1994) argued how different patterns of cognitive impairment mediate success of various operant learning methods based on memory load, comprehension of programme demands, and the degree of active (motor) participation required. They demonstrated, by taking these criteria into account, the successful reduction of aggressive behaviour shown by a patient who presented with very dense amnesia, using a particular operant learning intervention, response-cost (see Chapter 6). This work led to the development of a specific self-regulation intervention, self-monitoring training, and a neurobehavioural rehabilitation procedure for the management of challenging behaviour, including aggression, in the context of severe neurocognitive impairment. For detailed accounts of these methods see Alderman and Burgess (1994), Alderman (2003a), and Alderman, Wood and Worthington (2019).

Summary and conclusions

Aggression is arguably the most serious feature of NBD. Although prevalence varies, it is not uncommon, comprising a chronic condition that is capable of preventing rehabilitation and that can result in incarceration in inappropriate facilities. Primarily a product of neurological damage and neurocognitive impairment, aggressive behaviour is further shaped by a range of variables, including new learning, most notably an avoidance/escape or attention-motivated function. Methods from new learning theory have an excellent evidence base in the management of post-ABI aggression; the process model described earlier in this volume provides a framework to facilitate this. However, implementing a behaviour support plan requires caution if there is risk of physical assaults on others; when this is the case, it is recommended referral is made to NbR services. Other rehabilitation services can manage less risky aggressive behaviour; their capacity to do so is dependent on the degree to which they emulate the characteristics of NbR. To ensure conditions are as accommodating as possible to support new learning methods in behaviour support plans, the social climate should be person-centred, and the clinical team organised as a TDT.

Aggression creates a range of opinion within a team. Personal beliefs and attitudes underpin differences between members regarding the threshold beyond which it becomes categorised as problematic. Attributions regarding causation add to this variability. Some members may take it personally, others that it is an unmovable personality characteristic. Anxiety and fear further add to the mix. These factors undermine consistent delivery of behaviour support plans. Also, as seen with the case accounts above, learning can be slow, so perseverance is required. Sharing the formulation with all team members will go some way to depersonalise perceived motives of the aggressor. Getting everybody in the clinical team to agree behaviour is challenging and that it is in the best interests of the aggressor to change, is essential to ensure consistency of responses, Lack of consistency undermines treatment efficacy. When necessary, limiting the plan to a single task or session, implemented by a small subset of committed staff, demonstrates efficacy prior to wider use. With consistent delivery, the plan encourages team members to change their own behaviour and positively interact with the aggressor. Changing the behaviour of both the aggressor and their team undermines the reasons for aggression, as productive engagement in rehabilitation opens new doors and opportunities for people with ABI.

References

Alderman, N. (2001). Management of challenging behaviour. In R.Ll. Wood and T. McMillan (eds), *Neurobehavioural Disability and Social Handicap Following Traumatic Brain Injury*. Hove: Psychology Press.

Alderman, N. (2003a). Rehabilitation of behaviour disorders. In B.A. Wilson (ed.), *Neuropsychological Rehabilitation: Theory and Practice*. Lisse, The Netherlands: Swets and Zeitlinger.

Alderman, N. (2003b). Contemporary approaches to the management of irritability and aggression following traumatic brain injury. *Neuropsychological Rehabilitation*, *13*, 211–240.

Alderman, N. (2007). Prevalence, characteristics and causes of aggressive behaviour observed within a neurobehavioural rehabilitation service: Predictors and implications for management. *Brain Injury*, *21*, 891–911.

Alderman, N. (2015). Acquired brain injury, trauma and aggression. In G. Dickens, P. Sugarman and M. Picchioni (eds), *Handbook of Specialist Secure Care*. London: The Royal College of Psychiatrists.

Alderman, N. (2017). Interventions for Challenging Behaviour. In T. McMillan and R.Ll. Wood (eds), *Neurobehavioural Disability and Social Handicap Following Traumatic Brain Injury* (2nd edn). Abingdon: Psychology Press.

Alderman, N. and Burgess, P. (1994). A comparison of treatment methods for behaviour disorders following herpes simplex encephalitis. *Neuropsychological Rehabilitation, 4*, 31–48.

Alderman, N. and Groucott, L. (2012). Measurement of social climate within neurobehavioural rehabilitation services using the EssenCES. *Neuropsychological Rehabilitation, 22*, 768–793.

Alderman, N. and Knight, C. (1997). The effectiveness of DRL in the management and treatment of severe behaviour disorders following brain injury. *Brain Injury, 11*, 79–101.

Alderman, N., and Knight, C. (2017). Keeping the 'scientist-practitioner' model alive and kicking through service-based evaluation and research: Examples from neurobehavioural rehabilitation. *The Neuropsychologist, 3* (April), 25–32.

Alderman, N., Knight, C. and Morgan, C. (1997). Use of a modified version of the Overt Aggression Scale in the measurement and assessment of aggressive behaviours following brain injury. *Brain Injury, 11*, 503–523.

Alderman, N., Shepherd, J. and Youngson, H.A. (1992). Increasing standing tolerance and posture quality following severe brain injury using a behaviour modification approach. *Physiotherapy, 78*, 335–343.

Alderman, N., Williams, C. and Wood, R.Ll. (2021). Using the St Andrew's–Swansea Neurobehavioural Outcome Scale (SASNOS) to determine prevalence and predictors of neurobehavioural disability amongst survivors with traumatic brain injury in the community. *Neuropsychological Rehabilitation.* Advance online publication, 28 June 2021. https://doi.org/10.1080/09602011.2021.1946092

Alderman, N., Wood, R.Ll. and Williams, C. (2011). The development of the St Andrew's–Swansea Neurobehavioural Outcome Scale: Validity and reliability of a new measure of neurobehavioural disability and social handicap. *Brain Injury, 25*, 83–100.

Alderman, N., Wood, R.Ll. and Worthington, A. (2019). Environmental and behavioral management. In J.M. Silver, T.W. McAllister and D.B. Arciniegas (eds), *Textbook of Traumatic Brain Injury* (3rd edn). Washington, DC: American Psychiatric Publishing Inc.

Baguley, I.J., Cooper, J. and Felmingham, K. (2006). Aggressive behaviour following traumatic brain injury: How common is common? *Journal of Head Trauma Rehabilitation, 21*, 45–56.

Burgess, P.W. and Alderman, N. (1990). Rehabilitation of dyscontrol syndromes following frontal lobe damage: A cognitive neuropsychological approach. In R.Ll. Wood and I. Fussey (eds), *Cognitive Rehabilitation in Perspective.* Basingstoke: Taylor & Francis.

Dyer, K.F.W., Bell, R., McCann, J. and Rauch, R. (2006). Aggression after traumatic brain injury: Analysing socially desirable responses and the nature of aggressive traits. *Brain Injury, 20*, 1163–1173.

Eames, P.G. (2001). Distinguishing the neuropsychiatric, psychiatric, and psychological consequences of acquired brain injury. In R.Ll. Wood and T. McMillan (eds), *Neurobehavioural Disability and Social Handicap Following Traumatic Brain Injury.* Hove: Psychology Press.

Fazel, S., Lichtenstein, P., Grann, M. and Langstrom, N. (2011). Risk of violent crime in individuals with epilepsy and traumatic brain injury. *PloS Medicine, 8*, e10011050. http://journals.p;os.org/plosmedicine/artisle?id=10.1371/journal.pmed.1001150

Fleminger, S., Greenwood, R.J. and Oliver, D.L. (2006). Pharmacological management for agitation and aggression in people with acquired brain injury. *Cochrane Database Systematic Review, 4*, CD003299.

Gould, K.R., Hicks, A.J., Hopwood, M., Kenardy, J., Krivonos, I., Warren, N. and Ponsford, J. (2019). The lived experience of behaviours of concern: A qualitative study of men with traumatic brain injury. *Neuropsychological Rehabilitation, 29*, 376–394.

Kelly, G., Brown, S., Todd, J. and Kremer, P. (2008). Challenging behaviour profiles of people with acquired brain injury living in community settings. *Brain Injury, 27*, 457–470.

King, G., Strachan, D., Tucker, M., Duwyn, B., Desserud, S. and Shillington, M. (2009). The application of a transdisciplinary model for early intervention services. *Infants and Young Children, 22*, 211–223.

Legislation.gov.uk. (2015). Mental Health Act 1983. [online] Available at: http://www. legislation.gov.uk/ukpga/1983/20. [Accessed 27 February 2023].

Medd, J. and Tate, R.Ll. (2000). Evaluation of an anger management therapy programme following acquired brain injury: A preliminary study. *Neuropsychological Rehabilitation, 10*, 185–291.

Rahman, B., Oliver, C. and Alderman, N. (2010). Descriptive functional analysis of challenging behaviours shown by adults with acquired brain injury. *Neuropsychological Rehabilitation, 20*, 212–238.

Starkstein, S.E. and Robinson, R.G. (1991). The role of the human lobes in affective disorder following stroke. In H.S. Levin, H.M. Eisenberg and A.L. Benton (eds), *Frontal Lobe Function and Dysfunction* (pp. 288–303). Oxford: Oxford University Press.

Tam, S., McKay, A., Sloan, S. and Ponsford, J. (2015). The experience of challenging behaviours following severe TBI: A family perspective. *Brain Injury, 29*, 813–821.

Tateno, A., Jage, R.E. and Robinson, R.G. (2003). Clinical correlates of aggressive behavior after traumatic brain injury. *Journal of Neuropsychiatry and Clinical Neurosciences, 15*, 155–160.

Watson, C., Rutterford, N., Shortland, D., Williamson, N. and Alderman, N. (2001). Reduction of chronic aggressive behaviour ten years after brain injury. *Brain Injury, 15*, 1003–1015.

Williams, W.H., Mewse, A.J., Tonks, J., Mills, S., Burgess, C.N.W. and Cordan, G. (2010). Traumatic brain injury in a prison population: Prevalence, and risk for re-offending. *Brain Injury, 24*, 1184–1188.

Wood, R.Ll. (2001). Understanding neurobehavioural disability. In R.Ll. Wood and T. McMillan (eds), *Neurobehavioural Disability and Social Handicap Following Traumatic Brain Injury*. Hove: Psychology Press.

Wood, R.Ll. and Alderman, N. (2011). Applications of operant learning theory to the management of challenging behaviour after traumatic brain injury. *Journal of Head Trauma Rehabilitation, 26*, 202–211.

Wood, R.Ll., Alderman, N. and Worthington, A. (2020). Neurobehavioural rehabilitation. In N. Agrawal, R. Faruqui and M. Bodani (eds), *Oxford Textbook of Neuropsychiatry* (pp. 475–481). Oxford: Oxford University Press.

Ylvisaker, M., Turkstra, L., Coehlo, C., Yorkston, K., Kennedy, M., Sohlberg, M.M. and Avery, J. (2007). Behavioural interventions for children and adults with behaviour disorders after TBI: Systematic review of the evidence. *Brain Injury, 21*, 769–805.

9 What can behavioural interventions contribute to rehabilitation for inappropriate sexual behaviour post-acquired brain injury?

Caroline Knight

Introduction

Sexuality is a core element of human life influencing sense of self and expression in everyday actions, relationships with others and the world. It is 'with us from the moment of birth to the moment of death' (Zilbergeld, 2004). Quality of life is heavily influenced by the successful development and expression of adult sexuality (Blackerby, 1990). 'Sexuality is impacted in a myriad of ways following brain injury' (Ponsford, Downing and Stolwyck, 2017), including changes in motor control or sensation and pain, mediating the ability to engage in or take pleasure from sexual activity. Moreno et al. (2013) note that 'sexuality is closely tied to one's identity, self-esteem, and need for intimate relationships, all of which can be shaken after a traumatic brain injury'. Consequently, there can be changes in the libido and sexual preferences of an individual, in their capacity to give and receive love and affection and in the dynamics of existing partner relationships (e.g., Kreutzer and Zasler, 1989). This can be a particular concern when dealing with the many injuries that occur in children and young people, when sexuality is still developing, potentially arresting opportunities for future maturity.

The consequences appear widespread with 50 to 60 per cent of people reporting some level of disruption to their sexuality post-TBI (Moreno et al., 2013). Interviewing a large sample of people with moderate to severe TBI, Stolwyk et al. (2013) reported the following when compared to age- and gender-matched controls: significantly less importance attached to sexuality; reduced sex drive, enjoyment and sexual activity; and decreased ability to stay aroused, climax and give their partner sexual satisfaction.

Given the importance of sexuality in so many aspects of identity and relationships, sexual function and sexual behaviour deserves a central place within neurorehabilitation programmes. It is recommended that, due to the complex nature of related issues and interactions between factors, that a biopsychosocial framework be adopted. This chapter will review the neurological basis for sexual behaviour after acquired brain injury, its assessment and psychological approaches to management with the aid of case studies that illustrate the core principles discussed.

DOI: 10.4324/9781003083290-12

What is inappropriate sexual behaviour?

As a result of the complex mechanisms involved in acquired brain injury, changes in behaviour that could be construed as over-personal or inappropriately sexual occur in some individuals. These changes are attributable to the complex aetiology, including damage to the brain, particularly the frontal and temporal regions, that cause neurocognitive changes leading to reduced self-monitoring and empathy or reduced mental capacity to understand sexual relationships or the risks of expressed behaviours. Brain injury (frontal, medial temporal/limbic, diencephalic) can cause changes in (i) sex drive, (ii) sexual identity, (iii) sexual performance, and (iv) self-control. Emotional adjustment to the injury and psychosocial implications affecting the ability to express sexual needs may be contributing factors. Post-injury learning and environmental influences also play a role in the development and maintenance of new behaviours. The rehabilitation environment can also be a factor, increasing sexual frustration while minimising the opportunity for sexual expression.

ISB has received less attention than aggression as a challenging phenomenon post-injury, and, in their 2006 review, Johnson, Knight and Alderman argued that the limited published research reflected inconsistent terminology and subjective definitions being applied. Consequently, the authors offered a definition of ISB that has become more widely accepted: 'any verbal or physical act of an explicit or perceived sexual nature which is unacceptable within the social context in which it is carried out'.

When does ISB become challenging?

ISB is one of the most significant and pervasive neurobehavioural contributors to social handicap. Outcomes may involve social isolation, relationship breakdown, loss of employment and loss of independence and they may also attract criminal proceedings. Given the intimate and sensitive nature of sexual behaviour and relationships with partners, close relatives and friends may be put under immense strain as a direct result of ISB. Professional care staff are likely to experience ISB first-hand with as many as 70 per cent of brain injury rehabilitation professionals having reported sexual touching as a common problem within their facilities, and 20 per cent that identified sexual force as something commonly used by their patients in a study by Bezeau, Bogod and Mateer (2004).

Judgement of the appropriateness of behaviour will warrant careful thought, depending on the nature of the incident, environment, whether other person/s are the focus, awareness and intent involved, and who is present. Cultural norms and legislation vary considerably depending on where in the world issues occur and the values of local communities. Rehabilitation staff rating the severity of ISB in a UK rehabilitation setting cited touching of groins, breasts and buttocks as most intrusive and concerning (Knight, Alderman, Johnson, Green, Birkett-Swan and Yorston, 2008). However, in a replication of this study in Indonesia, discussed in a personal communication with the author, touching of the inner thigh was rated equally intrusive. Behaviours requiring further investigation and intervention within a rehabilitation setting are likely to be those that increase vulnerability, limit or delay access to community resources, and decrease the likelihood of attaining full rehabilitation potential (Alderman, 2001).

Prevalence and nature of ISB

A retrospective file review for inpatient and outpatient rehabilitation services for people with TBI in Australia identified 6.5 per cent of patients as having committed some form of sexual 'offence' (based on them having displayed touching, exhibitionism or overt sexual aggression) (see Simpson, Blaszczynski and Hodgkinson, 1999). A wider range of behaviours (verbal comments, non-contact behaviours, exposure, and touching others) were collated using the St Andrew's Sexual Behaviour Assessment in a UK neurobehavioural service and pilot data reported by Knight et al. (2008) demonstrated ISB exhibited by 43 per cent of patients with ABI over a 10-week period. In a subsequent and larger sample, Alderman, Knight and Birkett-Swan (2009) reported 42 per cent over three months, with just two people accounting for nearly half of the almost 700 recordings, and with verbal comments being the most prevalent. ISB occurred when the demands of the rehabilitation programme were lower, which may reflect a means of expressing sexual needs through seeking social engagement as opposed to more frequently recorded aggressive behaviours, which appeared to fulfil a predominantly escape or avoidance function during high-demand structured rehabilitation sessions. Simpson, Sabaz and Daher (2013) monitored 507 clients in Australia with severe TBI in a community-based brain injury rehabilitation programme. Using the Overt Behaviour Scale 8.9 per cent demonstrated ISB over the previous three months (57.9 per cent sexual talk, 29.8 per cent touching and 10.5 per cent exhibitionism/public masturbation). Almost all ISB occurred alongside other challenging behaviour (other aspects of social behaviour or aggression); and it was more likely in younger people and those with severe brain injury. In specialist neurobehavioural services, the suggested prevalence increases to around a quarter of cases (Kelly et al., 2022).

Differences in prevalence rates may reflect the recording tools adopted, described in detail in the assessment section of this chapter, as well as variation in cultural and service provision in the samples. However, it is unsurprising that higher levels of ISB were reported in inpatient neurobehavioural settings where more serious forms of ISB are a common reason for formal admission into hospital settings using relevant legislation, including the Mental Health Act (1983) [in England and Wales].

The question of 'intent'

Whether the behaviour observed is deliberately intended as a sexual act is a barrier to the identification of ISB disclosed by workers within neurorehabilitation (Knight et al., 2008) and other hospital settings (Hayward, Robertson and Knight, 2012). The limited opportunity for privacy in institutionalised settings and the fact that staff work in close physical proximity during personal care routines render recognition ambiguous. An open discussion of events, regardless of intention, can assist teams in differentiating accidental incidents (such as a hand brushing against the intimate body parts of a worker during a physical intervention) from patterns of ISB (where persistent touching of workers might indicate a misinterpretation of undressing as an invitation for sex).

Stigma and culture

How sexual behaviours are recognised or responded to is closely tied to the attitudes and values of the care staff (Lawrie and Jillings, 2004). Discomfort, embarrassment and denial around the sexual needs and behaviours of service users can lead to inflated or damaging attributions of risk or for sexual issues to be ignored completely (Ducharme and Gill, 1990; Zilbergeld, 2004; Johnson, Knight and Alderman, 2006; Hayward, Robertson and Knight, 2012). The neglect of sexual issues has implications for the well-being of those using the services and may be responsible for the evolution and maintenance of ISB, thereby compromising rehabilitation outcomes and leading to the potential burnout of staff. Clear boundaries and structured guidance within clinical environments are imperative in encouraging an appropriate expression of sexual needs and avoiding inconsistency, which may inadvertently reinforce ISB, or indeed in eradicating unethical responses, which could constitute malpractice. Addressing sexuality via education and training for both service users and staff encourages healthy and appropriate behaviours to be expressed within the rehabilitation community and enables episodes of ISB to be monitored and responded to optimally.

Rehabilitation

Detailed reviews of the advantages of a neurobehavioural model and the neurocognitive limitations of talking therapies for challenging behaviour in acquired brain injury (e.g., Alderman, Knight and Brooks, 2018) are described elsewhere in this book and apply in cases of ISB. The scope of this chapter is to focus primarily on behavioural interventions in cases of ISB, although other techniques will be included as important complements.

Formal assessment tools

Some tools incorporate ISB within a broader spectrum of behaviour. The Ryden Aggression Scale (Ryden, 1988), includes 'sexually aggressive behaviour', making obscene gestures, touching body parts of another person, hugging, intercourse or kissing. Two of the 29 items within the Cohen-Mansfield Agitation Inventory (Cohen-Mansfield, Marx and Rosenthal, 1989) refer to verbal and physical 'sexual advances', with expanded definitions and the ability to record the frequency and disruptiveness of these. A measure of sexual aggression for inpatients in a psychiatric setting was developed by Jones et al. (2007), with five levels of severity formulated from of interviews with staff, personal experiences of the authors and a review of clinical notes, though the psychometric properties were not tested. None of these scales were conceptualised for ABI nor did they enable the context within which behaviour took place to be captured.

The OBS (Kelly et al., 2006) was developed to record challenging behaviours displayed by people with ABI in community settings. The OBS comprises nine categories of behaviour, one of which is ISB. Behaviours included are sexual talk and touching (non-genital), exhibitionism and masturbation, touching (genital), and sexual assault/rape. It generates information by inviting an informant to consider frequency and severity over a three-month period. The St Andrew's Swansea Neurobehavioural Outcomes Scale (SAS-NOS) (Alderman, Wood and Williams, 2011) consists of 49 items measuring five principal domains of NBD generated by respondents rating frequency. Three items compose a sexual inhibition factor, including crude sexual comments, over-familiarity during social encounters, and touching self or others inappropriately. Both OBS and SASNOS were conceptualised for ABI, provide a profile of strengths and weaknesses, and have known psychometric properties, enabling valuable contributions to assessment, formulation and measuring outcome. The authors acknowledge threats to reliability and validity inherent in retrospective informant-based tools, as staff may not have witnessed or remembered all incidents of behaviour. There are also limitations in providing sufficient detail to conduct a functional analysis of behaviour.

Using the SASBA (Knight et al., 2008), observers record each episode of behaviour seen providing continuous measurement of ISB, and so it is less susceptible to observer error. The SASBA gathers data exclusively relevant to behaviour that could be construed as over-personal or inappropriately sexual dependent upon the context in which it occurs, and accordingly it collates setting events, antecedents and consequences of incidents that inform detailed functional or applied behaviour analysis. Moreover, it can facilitate review of the intrusiveness of interventions adopted to manage behaviour. Four categories of behaviour (verbal comments, non-contact, exposure and touching others) are included, each with four levels of severity, accompanied by detailed descriptors developed with reference to relevant literature and real examples of ISB reported by clinical staff. Staff rank items in order of severity following the definition offered by Kelly et al. (2006), 'the extent to which the behaviour might present a problem or concern, cause distress to staff and/or family, disrupt service delivery or interfere with social and community reintegration'. The SASBA has good inter-rater and test-retest reliability. It enables better-informed and evidence-based discussions about sexual behaviour, as well as conveying the relevance and importance of ISB when implemented.

Assessment and formulation

Thorough appreciation of the origins and function of ISB can only occur with wider scrutiny of the experiences of the individual and their surrounding context. Where possible, with consent, there should be discussion with the person and significant others. Dealing with sexual issues requires sensitivity in approach and careful thought about who in the clinical team is best placed to conduct interviews; indeed, there may need to be more than one therapist involved allocated to different parties. Limitations of confidentiality will vary depending on the circumstances, but this should be understood by all parties wherever possible. Box 9.1, whilst not exhaustive, details some of the relevant factors that may be relevant to explore.

Box 9.1   Factors that may be relevant to explore in the assessment of ISB

Neurological

- Brain injury (frontal, medial temporal/limbic, and diencephalic) can cause changes in (i) sex drive, (ii) sexual identity (iii) sexual performance, and (iv) self-control.

History

- likes, dislikes and preferences
- sexual health
- life story and experiences
- developmental
- trauma

Physical

- changes in experience
- pain, sensation
- drive, arousal, and ability to climax
- medications, alcohol or recreational drugs
- functional ability

Cognitive

- vulnerabilities
- insight and awareness
- self-monitoring
- empathy
- capacity issues in relation to specific issues

Psychological

- fears and anxieties
- depression
- self-esteem
- identity
- hopes, wishes and expectations

Systemic

- relationships and how values and wishes align
- opportunities
- freedom, choice
- privacy
- staff beliefs and perceptions, culture of service
- online and social networking
- exploitation and abuse

Once all relevant information has been collected, it is integrated to generate hypotheses about contributing or maintaining factors. The formulation process draws together information from multiple sources and is integrated with knowledge from the literature regarding ISB and ABI.

Context of intervention

Some authors have proposed that the implementation of intervention techniques for ISB be arranged in a hierarchy according to the severity of brain injury, degree of self-control and level of independence (Bezeau, Bogod, and Mateer, 2004; Moreno et al., 2013). For milder injuries, psychoeducation, social skills training and insight may be adopted, whereas, in severe ABI, interventions may encompass close supervision, establishment of boundaries, extinction of inappropriate behaviours and reinforcement of appropriate behaviours through conditioning.

Clinical teams may have a role in supporting a person's sexual functioning in clinical practice in a variety of ways, including providing sex and relationship education, considering masturbation and sex aids or pornography, or reviewing their opportunity to meet potential partners. These interventions must be considered within the limits of the legislation of relevant country (e.g. Mental Capacity Act, 2005 [in England and Wales]) and there will be other complex legal issues and professional standards that clinicians should operate within. These issues are discussed in detail in the British Psychological Society's guidance on capacity to consent to sexual relations (Herbert et al., 2019).

Furthermore, clinical teams should be mindful of systemic issues. Privacy and confidentiality may prove challenging. In circumstances where young adults have identified they would like to buy a sex aid to assist in masturbation but where their parents hold financial responsibility, careful negotiation on behalf of the clinician may be required both to secure the funding and to consider their client's potential reluctance to disclose the reasons for this. The same issue may arise where financial responsibility is invested in another party such as (in England and Wales) the Court of Protection. It may be appropriate to work together with individuals displaying ISB and their partners directly. People with ABI can also find themselves in relationships where they are the victim of ISB from others in their lives and may require support in navigating these difficulties and sexual vulnerabilities. Partners of people with ABI are likely to require time, space and possible access to their own therapy to adjust to changes in relationships.

Effectiveness of behavioural intervention

Earlier in this book the effectiveness of neurobehavioural rehabilitation programmes for challenging behaviour, including ISB, are reported (see also, for example, Wood and Alderman, 2011), as well as the merits of positive behavioural support and single case experimental design and as such will not be repeated here.

Several published SCEDs have described the successful reduction of ISB when behavioural interventions were employed; a combination of differential reinforcement of incompatible behaviours and time-out-on-the-spot (Alderman and Ward, 1991), differential reinforcement of low rates of behaviour (Alderman and Knight, 1997), and differential reinforcement of incompatible behaviour (Alderman, Knight and Brooks, 2013). ISB was also included within a targeted set of risky self-initiated verbal utterances via a five-stage process of self-monitoring training (Knight, Rutterford, Alderman and Swan, 2002).

Offensive sexual comments, touching of females (including genital areas) and public masturbation alongside aggression and coercion were the focus of another SCED in a male with severe ABI who was at risk of community services being withdrawn, criminal charges occurring or being admitted to a more restrictive institution (Kelly and Simpson, 2011). No baseline phase was included to compare subsequent phases of the design but strategies such as redirection, cueing appropriate behaviour and verbal feedback appeared to lead to some reduction in ISB. There were also facilitated visits to a sex worker in an attempt to support sexual expression which led to a further reduction in ISB. Legal, safety and ethical issues are explored by the authors and it is noted that these are likely to be country-dependent and the legalities of facilitated sex much more problematic in countries such as the UK.

Jan ter Mors, van Heughton and van Harten (2012) describe the reduction of ISB following the use of electrical aversion therapy in a 40-year-old man with TBI living with his mother. The ISB was said to be intrusive, including being directed towards a young child in the home on one occasion, though the nature and degree of these behaviours lack detail. They suggest all other treatment options had been exhausted, including non-aversive behavioural therapies, pharmacological interventions and admission into a mental health unit. This case has been included for the sake of completeness, but the ethical implications of the intervention are huge – rendering such an intervention highly controversial and outside of routine clinical practice governed by professional standards and legal authority in the UK.

In a group intervention, Kelly et al. (2022) report an exploratory clinical trial of community-based behaviour support interventions for ISB following ABI in the state of Victoria in Australia. Environmental change, psychoeducation and specific behavioural techniques were introduced for 24 individuals and behaviour data reflected significant decline using the OBS from baseline to closure and maintained at follow-up. Whilst this study did not control for specific interventions and there was some missing data, the authors argued the value of interventions employed in the naturalistic environment that targeted antecedent management and were multifocal and multimodal.

Case studies

Three case studies are presented as illustrations of a range of behavioural interventions in the treatment of ISB. Personal details have been altered to protect the identity of those involved.

Case 1: Feedback

Background

- GH was an 82-year-old man admitted from an acute hospital for a period of intensive neurorehabilitation following a second stroke, the first being five years earlier.
- Previously, GH had been living at home with a domiciliary care package to assist with personal care and all preparation of meals and domestic tasks.
- His right-sided weakness and spasticity had worsened and he now had no functional use of his right upper limb and was unable to bear weight.
- There was increased expressive dysphasia and verbal dyspraxia, and his speech deteriorated when he became tearful frequently throughout the day.
- GH sometimes refused to let go of female staff or pulled them towards him in an attempt to kiss them. He made physical gestures, blowing kisses and indicating their breasts, and he also touched their breasts and bottoms.

Assessment

- GH indicated feeling low, feelings of loneliness, and frustrations around his loss of independence and uncertainty around his future.
- He enjoyed spending time in the company of others in activities on the unit, especially when outdoors, and often discussed his love of gardening.

- GH was widowed many years earlier and had had no partner since. His daughters reported that he had displayed ISB towards the support workers who provided his care at home and as a result this was not an option to return to. They also said they knew he accessed online pornography at home.
- The referrer said the ISB was a barrier to finding a longer-term placement for him.
- Cognitive assessment highlighted his perseverance as a strength but suggested severe difficulties with finding the right words, concentration and memory and, whilst willing to try, he struggled to use his non-dominant left hand for writing or drawing.
- Use of the SASBA over a two-week period revealed 13 incidents of non-contact behaviours and touching others, including one severe incident of grabbing a staff member's breast. These took place within structured rehabilitation sessions and antecedents included being in close proximity to female staff or were prompted by verbal interaction. These behaviours were downplayed through the use of TOOTS.

Formulation

- GH used gesture and touch as a form of communication to supplement his verbal difficulties with speech. His touching of others was often appropriate to the social context (holding the hand of a staff member when upset) but could also become inappropriate, being unwilling to let go of staff or representing a sexual need. The function of the behaviour was suggested to be an expression of frustration and of the need to seek comfort. His behaviours were considered to be self-reinforcing resulting in some pleasure. The team were keen to understand if this process could be interrupted through feedback.

Intervention

- GH was encouraged to speak slowly and use gesture and an alphabet chart. He was given regular sessions with the team to listen and explore his concerns.
- Structured feedback in the form of a verbal prompt was implemented (e.g., 'That makes me feel uncomfortable') when episodes of ISB occurred.
- Arrangements were also made for GH to access his regular pornographic material at week 4.

Outcome

- Results are shown in Figure 9.1. It can be seen that SASBA recordings initially reduced following access to pornography but then increased again the following week. Recordings reduced significantly and were maintained at a lower level following the structured verbal feedback.
- As a result of the reduction in ISB, GH transferred to a care home close to his family for a longer-term placement. At the point of being discharged he could walk short distances and said he looked forward to accessing the greenhouse at the home and to the company of others.

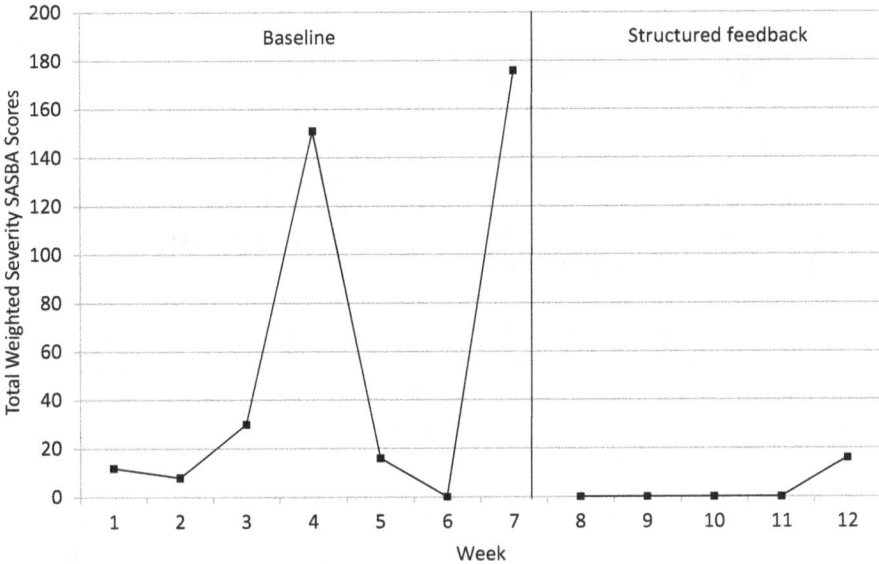

Figure 9.1 Total weighted severity of SASBA scores in response to the use of structured verbal feedback.

Case 2: Schedule of reinforcement

Background

- Aged 22, RF experienced a hypoxic brain injury.
- He had commenced his first job in a graduate scheme and lived a full social life with many friends, girlfriend and family close by.
- RF was fully mobile and able to eloquently express himself.
- His approach to activities of daily living was chaotic. He insisted he could complete all tasks independently but, if left to his own devices, he appeared unkempt, his surroundings were untidy and there was evidence of dyspraxia and sequencing difficulties when preparing snacks and doing his laundry.
- RF was keen to complete his rehabilitation quickly and return to his previous life.
- On admission to the unit, RF struggled with impulsivity and inhibitory control and made inappropriate verbal comments and touched others without their consent.

Assessment

- RF wanted others to 'talk to me like a normal person' and reported he 'hates being told what to do'. He found it difficult when he perceived boundaries being set by those he felt were 'younger', 'less intelligent' or with 'less in common' or if he sensed a 'lack of respect'. He enjoyed humour but sometimes his jokes were offensive to others. RF was aware that some tasks were now more effortful and formed negative appraisals, stating, for example, that he was 'stupid' and using other more abusive self-derogatory terms. He was desperate to get back to his job and to earning money.

- Relationships at home had become strained and members of his family reported he was unwilling to accept advice when his actions appeared risky or unsafe. His girlfriend had split up with him, and friends were reluctant to meet up due to his social behaviour including making offensive comments and contacting them at all hours.
- Neuropsychological assessment suggested his pre-morbid functioning was within the 'high average' range with his current cognitive functioning severely impaired. RF's language skills were well preserved, but his attention, memory and executive skills were significantly impaired.
- RF demonstrated verbal and physical aggression and, in addition, use of the SASBA highlighted verbal comments, non-contact behaviours and touching others. These occurred during structured activities and worsened when greater demands were placed upon him. Early warning signs included pacing behaviour and wandering away during conversations. Staff used TOOTS and activity distraction in order to manage his behaviours, but these were not always successful.

Formulation

- RF's ISB developed in the context of loss and adjustment to his ABI. Subsequent feelings of inferiority and anger led him to seek control over his situation and people around him. He craved the comfort and support of others, his opportunities for which had been curtailed as a result of ISB. His awareness and ability to self-monitor were limited and, as such, he failed to modify his behaviour and ISB was maintained. RF was vulnerable to retaliation from others and ISB was a barrier preventing his goal to move to a community setting. RF required an approach which would allow him to experience positive success in addressing his ISB.

Intervention

- A PBS plan was developed that included pro-active strategies such as phrasing advice positively and modifying the demands placed on RF, encouraging him to think through the benefits of tasks and his goals, and shaping his ISB into a more acceptable form such as giving a high five/fist bump.
- Psychological talking therapies were attempted, but RF found it difficult to sit still and became distracted by the environment when sessions were attempted walking outside. Some sessions needed to be discontinued as a result of him hugging and refusing to let go or throwing items at the psychologist 'as a joke'.

- A positive reinforcement schedule (DRI) programme was introduced where RF was offered daily verbal feedback and a tangible reinforcer of his choice (a small amount of money he could save and spend on items of his choice) contingent upon absence of inappropriate touching (as defined by any of the observable behaviours defined under the 'Touching Others' categories on the SASBA). He also completed a chart of his progress that he kept on his bedroom wall. RF was keen for the programme to commence, saying it would help him to achieve better control, and he was assessed to have capacity in relation to this decision.

Outcome

- Figure 9.2 shows a significant decline in touching behaviours specifically in response to DRI. By the time the intervention was withdrawn he had moved to a step-down community house. The gains made were maintained and also remained low at follow-up, approximately six months later, just prior to his discharge to a shared community house in his home area.
- Following discharge RF was able to fulfil his dream of returning to work, albeit in a less demanding field. He contacted the author to report the good news and reflected 'Really living life. My behaviour was biggest problem.'

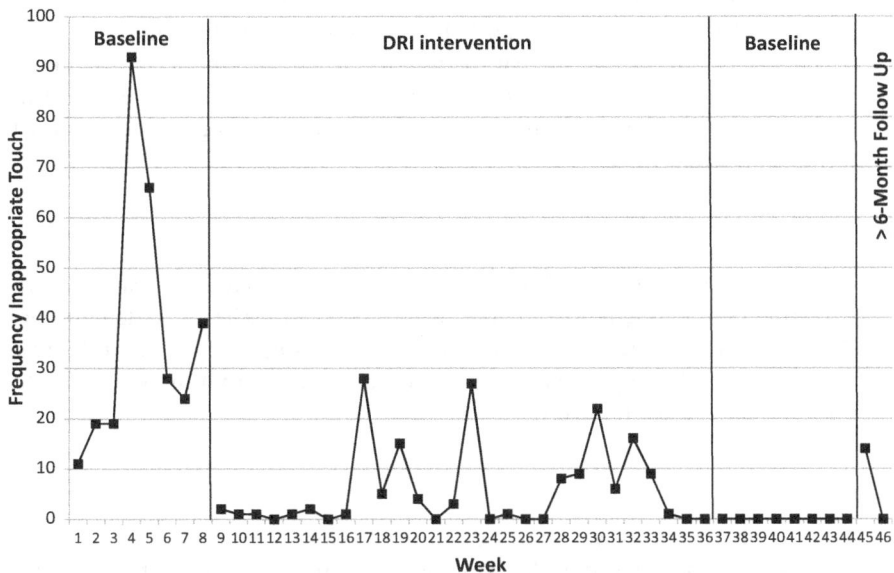

Figure 9.2 Response of inappropriate touching of other people to the use of differential reinforcement of incompatible behaviour.

Case 3: Response-cost

Background

- SN was in his late twenties when he experienced a road traffic accident resulting in a severe ABI with diffuse axonal injury. He was admitted to a post-acute facility and was assessed as being in post-traumatic amnesia for several weeks during which time he appeared confused and confabulated about why he was there.
- SN had lived independently close to his family home, worked in the leisure industry and had a series of girlfriends in the past. He enjoyed keeping fit and going on regular holidays abroad.
- SN required physiotherapy due to a high risk of falls and to work on his upper limb strength and coordination. He needed motivating to attend these sessions and prompts to remain focused on the task. He was easily distracted and made over-personal comments towards the therapist.

Assessment

- Following SN's emergence from PTA, there were ongoing and severe global cognitive difficulties demonstrated on assessment.
- SN described himself as 'not so shy, which is bad as women don't like it' and stated 'I wish my injury didn't happen, as it's put me back with women'.
- SN's family reported episodes of sexual comments made to members of the public when on home leave but also towards his sister-in-law who was distressed by this and had begun not to visit when he was there.
- Use of the SASBA identified that ISB was present from the point of admission and had lessened but there were ongoing verbal comments, non-contact behaviours and touching others directed towards male and female staff. ISB occurred in structured sessions and often followed verbal guidance to assist in the completion of a task.

Formulation

- SN missed the opportunity for intimate relationships but there was also evidence that ISB was used to avoid or escape from situations he found demanding.
- SN appeared unaware that ISB was consistently TOOTS by staff, and it was postulated that he required an approach that would help him build skills to self-monitor more effectively.

Intervention

- Baseline observations were carried out in physiotherapy sessions.
- SN was aware he sometimes 'makes comments to women that they may not like' including 'asking them to sleep with me'. He was deemed to lack capacity to make a decision to consent to a behavioural programme. His family

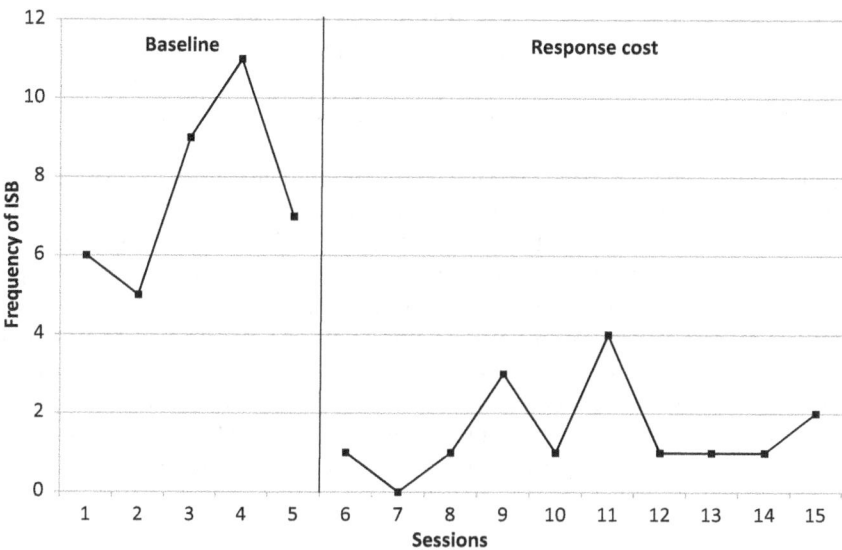

Figure 9.3 Effect of response-cost on frequency of inappropriate sexual behaviour in physiotherapy sessions.

and other professionals were involved in a best interest decision and a response-cost programme commenced (e.g., Alderman and Ward, 1991). SN received structured feedback about his ISB and received positive rein-forcement (he chose trips to the on-site café) at the end of the session, depending on the level of control over his behaviour. SN was given counters, which he was prompted to hand over when ISB occurred in order to improve self-monitoring of the behaviour.

Outcome

- Figure 9.3 highlights the decrease in frequency of ISB displayed following the introduction of response-cost.
- Response-cost was withdrawn as SN began spending much more time at home reducing the opportunities for the programme to run. He was dis-charged soon after with a 24-hour care package in his own home.
- By the time he discharged SN was mobilising independently.

Conclusions

ISB is relatively common following ABI, and it is optimally viewed from a biopsychosocial perspective considering the unique aspects of an individual's life and context as well as wider aspects of their sexual experience and needs. There are no universal answers in treatment as each person's unique neurobehavioural profile should be formulated from detailed assessment of the predisposing, contributing and maintaining factors. Behavioural interventions can be effective in treating ISB especially where there are challenges to using talking therapies or where insight and awareness are reduced. The complexity of capacity, consent, and ethical and legal issues need careful navigation. It is recommended that wherever possible clinicians endeavour to co-produce intervention plans collaboratively with people with ABI and the three case studies presented demonstrate this to varying degrees. ISB exists within a wider systemic context and involvement of significant others should also be an aspiration, though this will require mindful thought and need to be case-specific. In addition to behavioural interventions, clinicians can review how and if sexual expression can be facilitated appropriately and address the stigma that exists in services through staff education and training programmes. The SASBA may have a special role in empowering teams to notice ISB when it happens, ensure considered responses and give confidence to teams to discuss the associated issues more comfortably.

References

Alderman, N. (2001). Management of challenging behaviour. In R.Ll. Wood and T. McMillan (eds), *Neurobehavioural Disability and Social Handicap Following Traumatic Brain Injury*. Hove: Psychology Press.

Alderman, N. and Knight, C. (1997). The effectiveness of DRL in the management and treatment of severe behavioural disorders following brain injury. *Brain Injury*, *11*, 79–101.

Alderman, N., Knight, C. and Birkett-Swan, L. (2009). Inappropriate sexual behaviour and aggression observed within a neurobehavioural rehabilitation service: SASBA and OAS-MNR outcomes over a three-month period. *Journal of Cybertherapy and Rehabilitation*, *2*, 205–220.

Alderman, N., Knight, C. and Brooks, J. (2013). Rehabilitation approaches to the management of aggressive behaviour disorders after acquired brain injury. *Brain Impairment*, *14*, 5–20.

Alderman, N., Knight, C. and Brooks, J. (2018). Therapy for acquired brain injury. In A.R. Beech, A.J. Carter, R.E. Mann and P. Rotshtein (eds), *The Wiley Blackwell Handbook of Forensic Neuroscience*. Chichester: John Wiley and Sons.

Alderman, N. and Ward, A. (1991). Behavioural treatment of the dysexecutive syndrome: Reduction of repetitive speech using response cost and cognitive overlearning. *Neuropsychological Rehabilitation*, *1*, 65–80.

Alderman, N., Wood, R.Ll. and Williams, C. (2011). The development of the St Andrew's–Swansea Neurobehavioural Outcome Scale: Validity and reliability of a new measure of neurobehavioural disability and social handicap. *Brain Injury*, *25*, 83–100.

Bezeau, S.C., Bogod, N.M. and Mateer, C.A. (2004). Sexually intrusive behaviour following brain injury: Approaches to assessment and rehabilitation. *Brain Injury*, *18*, 299–313.

Blackerby, W.F. (1990). A treatment model for sexuality disturbance following brain injury. *Journal of Head Trauma Rehabilitation*, *5*, 73–82.

Cohen-Mansfield, J., Marx, M.S. and Rosenthal, A.S. (1989). A description of agitation in a nursing home. *Journal of Gerontology*, *44*, 77–84.

Ducharme, S. and Gill, K.M. (1990). Sexual values, training and professional roles. *Journal of Head Trauma Rehabilitation, 5*, 38–45.

Hayward, L., Robertson, N. and Knight, C. (2012). Inappropriate sexual behaviour and dementia: An exploration of staff experiences. *Dementia, 12*, 463–480.

Herbert, C., Joyce, T., Gray, G. and Betteridge, S. (2019). *Capacity to Consent to Sexual Relations*. Leicester: The British Psychological Society.

Jan ter Mors, B., van Heughton, C.M. and van Harten, P. (2012). Evaluation of electrical aversion therapy for inappropriate sexual behaviour after traumatic brain injury: A single case experimental design study. *BMJ Case Reports, 24*, 1–5.

Johnson, C., Knight, C. and Alderman, N. (2006). Challenges associated with the definition and assessment of inappropriate sexual behaviour amongst individuals with an acquired neurological impairment. *Brain Injury, 20*, 687–693.

Jones, N.T., Sheitman, B., Hazelrigg, M., Carmel, H., Williams, J. and Paesler, B. (2007). Development of a clinical instrument to record sexual aggression in an inpatient psychiatric setting. *Journal of Sexual Aggression, 13*, 51–58.

Kelly, G., Brown, S., Gillett, L., Descaller, J. and Simpson, G.K. (2022). Can behaviour support interventions successfully treat inappropriate sexual behaviour after acquired brain injury in community settings? A case series (N = 24). *Neuropsychological Rehabilitation, 32*, 407–428.

Kelly, G. and Simpson, G. (2011). Remediating serious inappropriate sexual behaviour in a male with severe acquired brain injury. *Sexuality Disability, 29*, 313–327.

Kelly, G., Todd, J., Simpson, G., Kremer, P. and Martin, C. (2006). The Overt Behaviour Scale (OBS): A tool for measuring challenging behaviours following ABI in community settings. *Brain Injury, 20*, 307–319.

Knight, C., Alderman, N., Johnson, C., Green, S., Birkett-Swan, L. and Yorston, G. (2008). The St Andrew's Sexual Behaviour Assessment (SASBA): Development of a standardised recording instrument for the measurement and assessment of challenging sexual behaviour in people with progressive and acquired neurological impairment. *Neuropsychological Rehabilitation, 18*, 129–159.

Knight, C., Rutterford, N.A., Alderman, N. and Swan, L.J. (2002). Is accurate self-monitoring necessary for people with acquired neurological problems to benefit from the use of differential reinforcement methods? *Brain Injury, 16* (1), 75–87.

Kreutzer, J.S. and Zasler, N.D. (1989). Psychosexual consequences of traumatic brain injury: Methodology and preliminary findings. *Brain Injury, 3*, 177–186.

Lawrie, B. and Jillings, C. (2004). Assessing and addressing inappropriate sexual behaviour in brain injured clients. *Rehabilitation Nursing, 29*, 9.

Moreno, J.A., Arango Lasprilla, J.C., Gan, C. and McKerral, M. (2013). Sexuality after traumatic brain injury: A critical review. *Neurorehabilitation, 32*, 69–85.

Ponsford, J.L., Downing, M. and Stolwyck, R. (2017). Sexuality and rehabilitation following acquired brain injury. In B.A. Wilson, J. Winegardener, C.M. van Heughton and T. Ownsworth (eds), *Neuropsychological Rehabilitation: An International Handbook*. Abingdon: Routledge.

Ryden, M.B. (1988). Aggressive behaviour in persons with dementia who live in the community. *Alzheimer Disease and Associated Disorders, 2*, 342–355.

Simpson, G., Blaszczynski, A. and Hodgkinson, A. (1999). Sex offending as a psychosocial sequela of traumatic brain injury. *Journal of Head Trauma Rehabilitation, 14*, 567–580.

Simpson, G.K., Sabaz, M. and Daher, M. (2013). Prevalence, clinical features, and correlates of inappropriate sexual behaviour after traumatic brain injury: A multicenter study. *Journal of Head Trauma Rehabilitation*, *28*, 202–210.

Stolwyk, R.J., Downing, M.G., Taffe, J., Kreutzer, J.S. Zasler, N.D. and Ponsford, J.L. (2013). Assessment of sexuality following traumatic brain injury: Validation of the Brain Injury Questionnaire of Sexuality. *Journal of Head Trauma Rehabilitation*, *28*, 164–170.

Wood, R.Ll. and Alderman, N. (2011). Applications of operant learning theory to the management of challenging behavior after traumatic brain injury. *Journal of Head Trauma Rehabilitation*, *26*, 202–211.

Zilbergeld, B. (2004). *Better than ever*. Bancyfelin: Crown House Publishing.

10 Managing behaviours that challenge in acute care settings

Alistair Teager and Abigail Methley

Acute care

Acute care within the United Kingdom's National Health Service (NHS) includes services such as accident and emergency (A&E) departments, inpatient and outpatient medicine, and surgery (The Health Foundation, 2020). It is designed to provide treatment for a severe injury, period of illness, urgent medical condition, or to recover from surgery. In essence, acute care is where a patient receives active, short-term treatment for a condition, such as in major trauma centres, hyperacute and acute stroke and neurorehabilitation, and critical care.

In terms of acquired brain injury, acute care settings may treat individuals in the early stages of recovery from traumatic brain injury, hypoxic brain injury or stroke; following neurosurgery as a result of subarachnoid haemorrhage (SAH), epilepsy or brain tumour; and also during the inpatient assessment or post-diagnosis of neurological issues such as encephalitis. These biological, cognitive and emotional changes may result in behaviours that are challenging for patients, families and staff to manage.

Common behaviours that challenge in acute settings

Whilst defining a behaviour as challenging to manage may be subjective and dependent on the context and available resources, common examples include: wandering/absconding, verbal aggression, physical aggression towards people and objects, self-harm, sexual behaviour that is inappropriate for the setting, low motivation, lying or confabulation, excessive complaining and demanding, stealing, and perseverative or repetitive behaviours. As well as common challenging-to-manage behaviours described in other chapters, some context-specific examples in acute settings include attempting to leave locked units, pulling out NG (nasogastric) and PEG tubes or tracheostomies, refusing to eat and drink, and refusing to take medication.

Inpatient neuropsychology referral data found that 'challenging behaviour' formed 7–13 per cent of referrals across hyperacute neurorehabilitation and stroke rehabilitation units (Watts and Teager, 2022; Khan-Bourne et al., 2017). These behaviours may be caused by physical, cognitive, psychological/

DOI: 10.4324/9781003083290-13

emotional or environmental/social factors. They may be due to sudden changes in mental state such as delirium or caused by a multitude of factors including severe or chronic illness, changes in metabolic balance (such as low sodium), medication, infection, surgery, psychiatric factors, such as psychosis, or alcohol/drug intoxication or withdrawal. They may relate to damage to specific areas of the brain, impacting emotional regulation or insight. They may also be caused by emotional responses to changes in physical health, the restrictions of rehabilitation settings, or exacerbation of pre-existing mental health conditions (e.g., psychosis, depression).

Behaviours that challenge can also arise from interpersonal conflict, often exacerbated by the interdependency present in acute settings (Hallett, 2018) and potentially by clashes of cultural responses and beliefs. This conflict can be with other staff, healthcare professionals, and patients and their families (Brinkert, 2010).

Below we outline a common presentation associated with challenging to manage behaviours in acute care settings.

Post-traumatic amnesia

Individuals commonly experience post-traumatic amnesia following TBI. PTA is defined as the time between a TBI and the return of continuous memory (Marshman et al., 2013). During this time, the injured person is conscious and awake, but is behaving or talking in a bizarre or uncharacteristic manner. The individual has no continuous memory of day-to-day events, and recent events may be equally affected, so that they are unable to remember what happened a few hours or even a few minutes prior.

The most obvious symptom is the loss of memory for the present time. The individual may recognise family and friends but be unable to process the fact that they are in hospital or have had an injury of some kind. Other common symptoms of PTA include:

- confusion, agitation, distress and anxiety;
- uncharacteristic behaviours such as violence, aggression, swearing, shouting, disinhibition;
- inability to recognise familiar people;
- tendency to wander.

In some cases, however, people may be very quiet, docile, loving and friendly. Length of PTA is linked to severity of TBI, and increased severity of TBI is associated with reduced prognosis (Baum et al., 2016; Ponsford, Spitz and McKenzie, 2016). A broad recovery process from PTA can be seen in Figure 10.1.

It is important to note that 30–70 per cent of patients admitted to acute rehabilitation, experience 'post-traumatic agitation' (Mortimer and Berg, 2017), and 41 per cent of patients with TBI on an acute hospital ward exhibited agitated behaviour during their stay (McNett, Sarver, and Wilczewski,

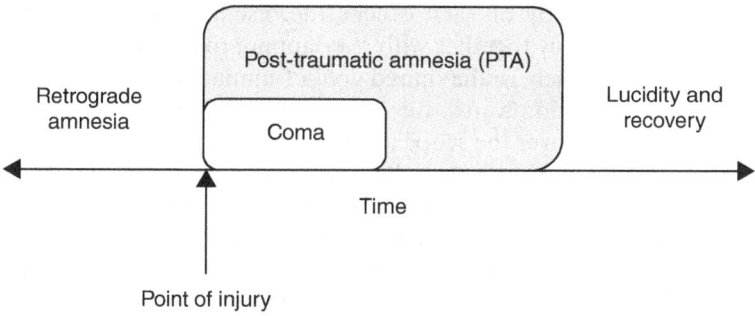

Figure 10.1 PTA recovery process.

2012). Agitation is associated with increased length of stay, reduced engagement in rehabilitation, less cognitive and motor recovery, and poorer functional outcomes as a result (McNett, Sarver and Wilczewski, 2012; Bogner et al., 2015; Nott, Chapparo and Baguley, 2006).

Post-neurosurgery

Similarly, recovery from neurosurgery (e.g., tumour removal, stopping brain haemorrhages, clot removal, aneurysm repair) can all lead to behaviours that challenge. The individual may be in the early stages of recovering from the neurosurgery itself, experiencing changes in cognition, behaviour, and emotion as a result of acute neurological changes or delirium, or from feelings of disorientation. There is little research on the consequences of challenging behaviours in conditions other than TBI, but it is reasonable to assume that it would detrimentally affect the patient journey, engagement in therapy and outcomes.

Summary

Early intervention within acute care settings is key to maximising recovery. For physical health this may relate to maximising the recovery window of opportunity where the maximum gain is seen. In psychological terms, early intervention may provide people with helpful frameworks to explain their difficulties in a positive way and may provide basic strategies to prevent mood-related issues increasing and becoming entrenched. Acute care settings therefore have the opportunity to provide positive early interventions for challenging behaviours that can emerge in the initial phase following an ABI.

The role of the interdisciplinary team

There are multiple models of care through which professionals from different disciplines work together to provide complex rehabilitation (Pelser, Banks and Bavikatte, 2023). Multidisciplinary teams (MDTs) are where each professional team works independently of each other. Interdisciplinary teams are where professionals work closely together with overlapping roles and responsibilities. As this applies most closely to the shared goal of managing challenging behaviour on acute rehabilitation wards, we will refer to IDTs in this chapter.

It is not possible to cover the scope of the extended IDT within this chapter (for two very helpful overviews see: Pelser, Banks and Bavikatte, 2023; and Elbaum, 2019). Key members include the consultant in rehabilitation medicine, rehabilitation specialist nurse, clinical psychologist/neuropsychologist, speech and language therapist, physiotherapist and occupational therapist, and additional specialisms include dieticians, pharmacists and many others. Some of the ways in which these professionals might play a part in managing challenging behaviours in acute settings are described in Figure 10.2.

Gillespie et al. (2017) explored IDT perceptions of the role of clinical neuropsychology and found that working with challenging behaviour and providing staff training and supervision were both rated as 7.8 out of 10 in terms of importance. This was lower than 'traditional' roles associated with

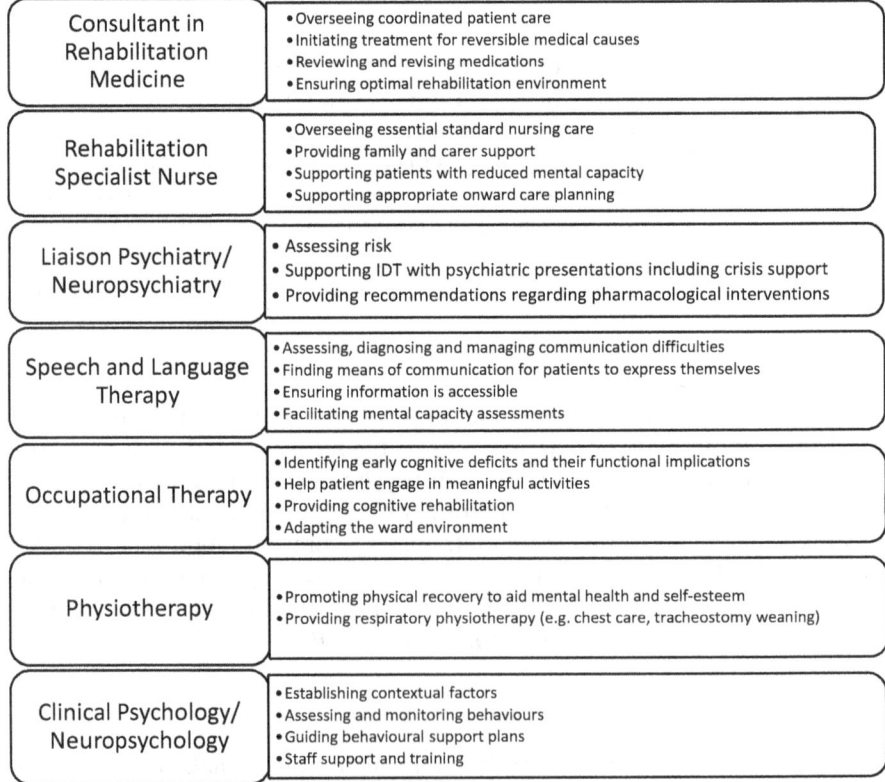

Figure 10.2 IDT roles in managing challenging behaviours in acute settings.

neuropsychology, such as assessing cognitive functioning (9.3), cognitive rehabilitation (9.2) and supporting emotional adjustment (8.6). This may represent perceived value, but with neuropsychology input in acute settings often limited or scarce, it may also be that working with challenging behaviours is not possible, and is therefore perceived to be of less importance. This has been alluded to by Soreny (2009), who found that nursing staff felt frustrated at their lack of 'mental health skills' when working with individuals displaying challenging behaviours in an acute care setting. Improving neuropsychology provision in acute settings is therefore of paramount importance in order to be able to improve outcomes for individuals who experience challenging behaviour following ABI and to fully support staff teams.

Evidence regarding managing challenging behaviours in acute settings

Despite the high prevalence of challenging behaviour within acute settings, there is a paucity of literature addressing its management. Hallett (2018) describes a framework outlining primary, secondary and tertiary levels of prevention to target (shown in Figure 10.3), while also recommending the opportunity for positive responses to challenging behaviours be supported at a strategic level.

Block et al. (2023) present a systematic review that summarises clinical practice guidelines outlining the assessment and management of challenging behaviour after moderate to severe TBI in adults within acute settings. The highest quality guidelines reviewed recommended comprehensive assessment is followed by non-pharmacological approaches and then by pharmacological approaches if required (Scottish Intercollegiate Guidelines Network, 2013; Bayley et al., 2016).

Evidence for non-pharmacological management of challenging behaviour

Literature suggests that non-pharmacological approaches, such as psychological interventions, may be moderately effective in reducing challenging

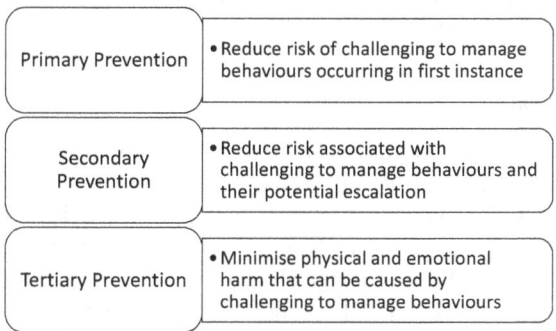

Figure 10.3 Prevention framework (Hallet, 2018).

behaviours within ABI, such as aggression (Byrne and Coetzer, 2016). Within the Block et al. (2023) guidelines review, the strongest supporting evidence base for non-pharmacological management in acute settings was for behaviour management plans incorporating positive behaviour interventions. In addition to the models already described within this textbook, the Newcastle model has a growing body of evidence (James and Jackman, 2017). It is a non-pharmacological approach that uses a biopsychosocial formulation to guide interventions designed to meet previously unmet needs. Whilst the main use of this model has been with people with dementia, including the management of challenging behaviours, it is similar in scope to alternative biopsychosocial approaches used within brain injury services. A core aspect is that it is systemic in nature, incorporating not just patient factors but also care-giver responses.

Evidence for pharmacological management of challenging behaviour

Pharmacological management of challenging behaviour includes the use of medication to address underlying medical conditions (e.g., the use of antibiotics for infections; thiamine for people with alcohol dependence), health needs (including medication to aid sleep) and mental health needs (including psychiatric medications). For the management of these behaviours more specifically, medications including anti-psychotics, antidepressants, mood stabilisers and sedatives are used.

In the Block et al. (2023) review, pharmacological interventions related predominantly to the management of agitation, aggression and impaired attention/arousal. The highest level of supporting evidence was for beta-blockers for aggression, selective serotonin re-uptake inhibitors for moderate agitation and irritability, and central nervous system stimulants and adamantanes for impaired arousal and attention. Expert-opinion-level recommendations were available for the pharmacological treatment of severe acute agitation and agitation of a level that threatened staff and patient safety. A need was identified for further rigorous research to determine the efficacy of pharmacological treatments on TBI agitation and aggression and to identify the most appropriate and validated behaviour management approach for challenging behaviours after TBI in acute settings.

Systemic considerations

In Block et al. (2023) the model of care was found to be very important, with strong supporting evidence for specialised TBI behaviour management provided through an MDT. There was expert-opinion-level evidence for education and training for healthcare professionals and education and contribution to feedback on behavioural data for people with TBI and their families. Previous research has also demonstrated the benefits of staff support including Balint groups for staff (Smart and Teager, 2018) or the use of structured staff forums, such as Schwartz Rounds.

Clinical case example

The following section aims to provide a hypothetical case example of challenging behaviours that are commonly seen in acute hospital settings. The approaches taken in this example will have a number of transferable or generalisable approaches for individuals with different diagnoses.

Tony: Traumatic brain injury

Background

Tony, 78, fell from a ladder while doing some house maintenance. He was admitted to the nearest major trauma centre (MTC) where a CT (computerised tomography) scan found that he had sustained a TBI. As Tony became more conscious, he was behaving and talking in a way his family felt were out of character and challenging for staff to manage. On the major trauma ward, Tony was swearing at staff, agitated and wandering. He appeared to forget information quickly and he struggled to recall what staff were saying to him or what had happened to him. The IDT found some important information in Tony's hospital notes, which indicated that he had high levels of agitation, identified infection, that it was a short time since admission, and that he had been prescribed antipsychotics to manage challenging behaviours. These have all be found to be covariates in challenging to manage behaviours (McKay et al., 2020).

The IDT were able to rule out other causes, and recognised Tony's presentation as post-traumatic amnesia following a TBI. Tony's age was of particular importance as older age can have a significant impact on emergence from PTA (Chua et al., 2012), and therefore on challenging behaviours. The IDT sought psychological support from the neuropsychology team, in line with the principles of stepped psychological care (Kneebone, 2016).

Assessment

An approach based on the principles of positive behavioural support was utilised for this case (Lavigna and Willis, 2005). Occupational therapists and neuropsychologists established his cognitive and functional baseline from his family. Prior to the fall, Tony was independent and had no cognitive issues. The IDT began to assess Tony's emergence from PTA formally using the Westmead post-traumatic amnesia (WPTA) scale (Marosszeky et al., 1997) to help understand emergence from PTA, which can be difficult to determine (Tate et al., 2006). The WPTA scale includes seven orientation items and five recall items. When combined with observational information from staff and family, an individual is usually felt to have 'emerged' from PTA when they score 12/12 on three consecutive days, but clinicians would be mindful of other influential factors (e.g., pre-admission diagnoses, length of time since WPTA commenced). The initial WPTA score was 4 out of 7, confirming his level of disorientation. Low initial PTA scores have been associated with more protracted emergence from PTA (Chua et al., 2012). The WPTA was administered daily to monitor progress. Behavioural observations were used to triangulate the IDT's opinion as to the challenges they were facing, as these complement memory-based PTA assessments in determining emergence from PTA (Weir et al., 2006), as well as providing valuable information about the presenting problems. The Agitated Behaviour Scale (ABS) (Corrigan, 1989) and sleep charts were utilised, completed by clinical support workers (CSWs) caring for Tony.

The ABS comprises 14 items, each rated using a 1–4 Likert scale. It allows IDTs to understand the frequency and intensity of the challenging behaviours, measure change and build behavioural support plans. Evidence-based alternative, or supplemental, observational measures that would be appropriate in an acute setting would include the Overt Aggression Scale – Modified for Neurorehabilitation (Alderman, Knight and Morgan, 1997) and the St Andrew's–Swansea Neurobehavioural Outcome Scale (Alderman, Wood and Williams, 2011).

The ABS data was gathered over three days and analysed by an assistant psychologist, who noted that Tony was sleeping three hours per night. Tony's total ABS score was 32 out of 56, falling within the 'moderate' range of agitation. The types of agitated behaviours that were presenting as challenging to the IDT centred around 'wandering from treatment areas', being 'uncooperative, resistant to care, demanding', and 'short attention span, easy distractibility, inability to concentrate'. The assistant psychologist and neuropsychologist therefore sought to gather more information about this using ABC charts. They did this by talking to IDT members working frequently and/or intensely with Tony to see if they could identify particular antecedents, behaviours and consequences therein. These ABC charts enabled the IDT to identify that challenging Tony verbally when he was wandering, or trying to leave the ward, resulted in Tony's agitation levels increasing and led him to become even more 'uncooperative'. In addition to this, it was found that when team members tried to help Tony with personal care, he became 'resistant to care' and verbally aggressive.

Tony's mental capacity to decide about remaining in hospital was assessed as he met the 'acid test' threshold for Deprivation of Liberty Safeguards in that, because of the TBI, he was under constant supervision and not free to leave (Department of Health, 2015). It was felt that he lacked the ability to make that specific decision at that time. A best interests meeting (BIM) was held, and it was agreed that the least restrictive option would be to keep him on a locked ward, initially with 24-hour supervision. As a result of this a Deprivation of Liberty Safeguard was requested (Mental Health Act, 2007).

Interventions

Based on the assessment information and acknowledging the limited evidence-base regarding managing challenging behaviours in acute settings (Block et al., 2023), Tony's behavioural support plan drew upon principles of primary, secondary and tertiary prevention (Hallett, 2018) embedded within a PBS framework.

Proactive strategies

The following strategies were implemented to try to prevent challenging behaviours arising.

ECOLOGICAL STRATEGIES/ENVIRONMENTAL MANAGEMENT

For Tony, this included moving him to a side room to reduce stimulation and trying to re-establish his sleep-wake cycle by ensuring that curtains were opened or closed, and lights were turned on or off, depending on time of day. Discussing potential pharmacological options to improve circadian rhythms was also explored with Tony's medical team (e.g., melatonin).

The IDT provided information on PTA and challenging behaviours to Tony's family to improve their understanding, and therefore help the IDT support Tony. As a part of the discussions with family, the IDT attempted to find out ways in which they might improve the way they interacted with Tony so that he might respond better to perceived authority, something that can affect challenging behaviours in PTA (Thomas, 2009). The nursing team also attempted to support Tony with one-to-one care from clinical support workers, whom he seemed to prefer, in order to reduce triggers for challenging behaviours, or their consequences.

POSITIVE PROGRAMMING/SKILLS TRAINING

Although still in PTA, it was felt appropriate to request a communication assessment from a speech and language therapist (Steel et al., 2015; Steel et al., 2017), given the foci of the TBI and the potential difficulties Tony had in communicating his needs, leading to challenging behaviours. The speech and language therapy (SALT) assessment highlighted cognitive communication difficulties and recommendations were provided in terms of best practice, including active listening techniques.

Orientation information was placed in Tony's room, and updated on a daily basis, in line with a North Star Project approach, as this has been found to be beneficial in terms of reducing length of PTA, increasing patient interactions and increasing family involvement (Thomas et al., 2003; De Guise et al., 2005). This was combined with repeated WPTA assessments to monitor orientation and emergence from PTA.

To improve independence, and reduce the need for support from staff, the IDT tried to help 'retrain' Tony's activities of daily living (Mortimer et al., 2019; Trevena-Peters, McKay and Ponsford, 2017), As a part of this, they utilised targeted Goal Attainment Scale (GAS) goals to challenge beliefs regarding therapy, build rapport and engagement, and catalyse progress (Trevena-Peters, McKay and Ponsford, 2017; Trevena-Peters, McKay and Ponsford, 2019). This was utilised in Tony's case in order to try to reduce the length of PTA, and chance of challenging behaviours therein. Activities of daily living retraining was used despite concerns about challenging behaviours, as this approach has not been found to increase agitation levels with patients in PTA (Trevena-Peters, Ponsford and McKay, 2018), but has been found to reduce the length of inpatient stay, readmission rates and the use of other medications. As a part of this, it was recognised that Tony would benefit from an early referral for acute neurorehabilitation, which has been linked to quicker emergence from PTA (Chua et al., 2012), and therefore fewer challenging behaviours.

FOCUSED SUPPORT/REINFORCEMENT STRATEGIES

Initially, Tony was supported on a one-to-one basis by IDT members who had undertaken person-centred training and e-learning provided by their service in managing challenging behaviours.

As a part of this, the IDT members utilised positive reinforcement to increase the frequency of more 'desirable' behaviours, such as engaging in care or therapy, or talking in an appropriate way to staff. In conjunction with this, the IDT used principles of negative reinforcement to reduce the frequency of challenging behaviours; these came in the form of sensitive verbal references to the challenging behaviour, with suggestions as to what a more desirable behaviour would look like. This approach can be useful when the individual is not able to engage in reasoned discussions about their actions (Matthies, Kreutzer and West, 1997). When the challenging behaviour desisted, the IDT provided specific positive reinforcement to acknowledge and validate this.

Reactive strategies

The aims of these strategies were to deal with challenging behaviours as they were continuing, with the main technique utilised being de-escalation (Hallett, 2018). Broad recommendations around physical and pharmacological interventions are also provided.

DE-ESCALATION

The IDT used de-escalation techniques when these were needed and they were delivered, where possible, by members of staff that knew Tony best (Yuen and Benzing, 1996; Matthies, Kreutzer and West, 1997). There were times when some degree of concession to Tony's demands was necessary, when safe and practical to implement.

PHYSICAL AND PHARMACOLOGICAL INTERVENTIONS

When Tony's challenging behaviours led to imminent risk of harm to self, others or property, and all other methods had been tried without success, the IDT utilised physical and/or pharmacological means of intervening as a last resort and the least restrictive options to meet the needs of the situation, in line with Deprivation of Liberty Safeguards (Mental Health Act, 2007).

Physical interventions might include providing one-to-one support or the use of locked doors on wards, for example, but it can also involve physical restraint. It was important that the acute hospital had a policy on physical interventions and pharmacological management of patients with acute neurological conditions that took into account various medical and neurological needs (Nash et al., 2019) and also that IDT members were trained in delivering them. In Tony's case, seeking advice from the treating team and experts within the acute hospital was vital (e.g., psychiatry, neurology, geriatrics).

FAMILY AND STAFF SUPPORT

In addition to the aforementioned interventions, it was also important to offer Tony's family support in terms of understanding common consequences of TBI, including challenging behaviours, and to provide emotional support for them in coping with the changes they were seeing as a result of his injury.

Furthermore, IDT members were supported by reflective practice sessions in the form of Balint groups.

The role for digital innovation

The use of digital health technologies (DHTs) within acute settings offers the opportunity to improve the understanding and management of challenging behaviours by providing the IDT with the right information at the right time. Digital methods of real-time data capture were not routinely used at the time the IDT supported Tony. However, they now offer great potential.

One example of this is Melo™ – a new artificial intelligence-driven (AI-driven) platform for clinicians to better capture and understand challenging behaviours. Developed by tech-for-good company Decently (www. decently.co.uk) – in collaboration with a number of NHS Trusts – Melo seeks to improve the understanding of both proactive (pre-incident) and reactive (post-incident) behaviours through its simple, yet powerful, app. An IDT can use Melo to collate meaningful data in real-time via a number of recognised assessment tools – standardising and streamlining the approach to collection of data. IDTs and other clinicians benefit from a range of data visualisations (e.g., graphs and charts) to identify trends, escalating patterns of behaviour and opportunities to personalise interventions for a patient.

This is currently undergoing a real-world validation in partnership with Salford Royal hospital (part of the Northern Care Alliance NHS Foundation Trust), where it will be trialled on two acute neurorehabilitation wards over a 12 month period. The longer-term goal is to be able to deploy Melo in a wide variety of settings and to grow and adapt the clinical content in order to be able to support patients with a variety of medical conditions (e.g., dementia, delirium, post-traumatic stress disorder (PTSD), etc.).

A full independent evaluation of the project will be undertaken by Manchester Metropolitan University and published in early 2024, however the potential benefits of embedding an ethical AI/digital first approach (like Melo) into daily patient care include the opportunity to:

1 improve patient outcomes via better prognosis, reduced length of stay, increased cognitive and motor recovery;
2 create a safer working environment for healthcare professionals by empowering staff to have a greater understanding of patient risks and needs;
3 support healthcare professionals to handle increased workload and reduce stress;
4 minimise observational and diagnostic errors through improved consistency and standardisation;
5 give time back to care givers to focus on more complex cases by streamlining and speeding-up of assessments.

Ultimately, digital health innovations like Melo have the potential to drive improved outcomes by making behavioural data more accessible and actionable, thus enabling healthcare professionals to make evidence-based decisions at critical steps of the patient journey.

Summary

Overall, a fixed/flexible approach to assessment was utilised with Tony, who had sustained a TBI. Preventative practice (Hallett, 2018) and PBS (LaVigna and Willis, 2005) were used as foundations for interventions, tailored to meet the needs of the individual. Considerations around training and support for families and staff, including the future potential for digital innovation were also described.

Summary and conclusions

Working with challenging behaviours in acute hospital settings is difficult due to the variable, dynamic nature of the presenting problems, and the impact these can have on staff morale, well-being and sickness and absence. Whilst guidelines for psychological, physical and pharmacological interventions do now exist, the quality of the evidence base is variable and further research is required, from single case experimental designs through to randomised controlled trials (RCTs). Commonly used approaches to managing challenging behaviours in other settings can be adapted and adopted in the acute environment, such as PBS (LaVigna and Willis, 2005) and the Newcastle Model (James and Jackman, 2017), and a clinical case example was provided describing how these could be done.

Recommended resources

Free to download posters on working with challenging to manage behaviours: https:// www.gmneurorehab.org.uk/educational-materials/

Mental Capacity (Amendment) Act, 2019. London: Her Majesty's Stationery Office.

References

Alderman, N., Knight, C. and Morgan, C. (1997). Use of a modified version of the Overt Aggression Scale in the measurement and assessment of aggressive behaviours following brain injury. *Brain Injury*, *11*, 503–523.

Alderman, N., Wood, R.Ll. and Williams, C. (2011). The development of the St Andrew's–Swansea Neurobehavioural Outcome Scale: Validity and reliability of a new measure of neurobehavioural disability and social handicap. *Brain Injury*, *25*, 83–100.

Baum, J., Entezami, P., Shah, K. and Medhkour, A. (2016). Predictors of outcomes in traumatic brain injury. *World Neurosurgery*, *90*, 525–529. https://doi.org/10.1016/j. wneu.2015.12.012

Bayley, M., Swaine, B., Lamontagne, M.E., Marshall, S., Allaire, A.S., Kua, A. and Marier-Deschênes, P. (2016). *INESSS-ONF Clinical Practice Guideline for the Rehabilitation of Adults with Moderate to Severe Traumatic Brain Injury*. Toronto: Ontario Neurotrauma Foundation. Available from: https://braininjuryguidelines.org/modtosevere/

Block, H., Paul, M., Muir-Cochrane, E., Bellon, M., George, S. and Hunter, S.C. (2023). Clinical practice guideline recommendations for the management of challenging behaviours after traumatic brain injury in acute hospital and inpatient rehabilitation settings: a systematic review. *Disability and Rehabilitation*, 1–11. https://doi.org/1 0.1080/09638288.2023.2169769

Bogner, J., Barrett, R.S., Hammond, F.M., Horn, S.D., Corrigan, J.D., Rosenthal, J., Beaulieu, C.L., Waszkiewicz, M., Shea, T., Reddin, C.J., Cullen, N., Giuffrida, C.G., Young, J. and Garmoe, W. (2015). Predictors of agitated behavior during inpatient rehabilitation for traumatic brain injury. *Archives of Physical Medicine and Rehabilitation*, *96* (8), Supplement, S274–S281. https://doi.org/10.1016/j.apmr.2015.04.020

Brinkert, R (2010). A literature review of conflict communication causes, costs, benefits and interventions in nursing. *Journal of Nursing Management*, *18* (2), 145–156.

Byrne, C. and Coetzer, R. (2016). The effectiveness of psychological interventions for aggressive behavior following acquired brain injury: A meta-analysis and systematic review. *NeuroRehabilitation*, *39* (2), 205–221.

Chua, K., Yap, S., Low, W. and Kong, K.H. (2012). Clinical and functional predictors of emergence from post traumatic amnesia (PTA) during inpatient rehabilitation for severe traumatic brain injury. *Brain Injury*, *26* (4–5), 572.

Corrigan, J.D. (1989). Development of a scale for assessment of agitation following traumatic brain injury. *Journal of Clinical and Experimental Neuropsychology*, *11*, 261–277.

De Guise, E., Leblanc, J., Feyz, M., Thomas, H. and Gosselin, N. (2005). Effect of an integrated reality orientation programme in acute care on post-traumatic amnesia in patients with traumatic brain injury. *Brain injury*, *19* (4), 263–269.

Department of Health (2015). *Department of Health Guidance: Response to the Supreme Court Judgment/ Deprivation of Liberty Safeguards*. https://assets.publishing. service.gov.uk/government/uploads/system/uploads/attachment_data/file/485122/ DH_Consolidated_Guidance.pdf

Elbaum, J. (2019). *Acquired Brain Injury: An Integrative Neuro-Rehabilitation Approach*. New York: Springer.

Gillespie, D.C., Alford, M., Young, L. and Gillanders, S. (2017). Staff perceptions of clinical neuropsychological work, and self-rated psychological skills and confidence, in the acute neuroscience setting. *The Neuropsychologist, 3*, 40–45.

Hallett, N. (2018). Preventing and managing challenging behaviour. *Nursing Standard, 32* (26), 51–63.

The Health Foundation (2020). *Acute Care*. https://www.health.org.uk/topics/acute-care

James, I. and Jackman, L. (2017). *Understanding Behaviour in Dementia that Challenges: A Guide to Assessment and Treatment* (2nd edn). London: Jessica Kingsley.

Khan-Bourne, N., Bancroft, V., Doyle, C., Morris, R. (2017). Neuropsychological rehabilitation in stroke care: A review of referrals and interventions offered across two stroke units. *The Neuropsychologist, 3*, 33–39.

Kneebone, I.I. (2016). Stepped psychological care after stroke. *Disability and Rehabilitation, 38* (18), 1836–1843.

LaVigna, G. and Willis, T. (2005). A positive behavioural support model for breaking the barriers to social and community inclusion. *Tizard Learning Disability Review, 10* (2), 16–23. https://doi.org/10.1108/13595474200500016

Marosszeky, N.E.V., Ryan, L., Shores, E.A., Batchelor, J. and Marosszeky, J.E. (1997). *The PTA Protocol: Guidelines for Using the Westmead Post-Traumatic Amnesia (PTA) Scale*. Sydney: Wild and Wooley.

Marshman, L.A., Jakabek, D., Hennessy, M., Quirk, F. and Guazzo, E.P. (2013). Post-traumatic amnesia. *Journal of Clinical Neuroscience, 20* (11), 1475–1481. https://doi.org/10.1016/j.jocn.2012.11.022

Matthies, B.K., Kreutzer, J.S. and West, D.D. (1997). *The behavior management handbook: A practical approach to patients with neurological disorders*. Tucson, AZ: Therapy Skill Builders.

McKay, A., Love, J., Trevena-Peters, J., Gracey, J. and Ponsford, J. (2020). The relationship between agitation and impairments of orientation and memory during the PTA period after traumatic brain injury. *Neuropsychological Rehabilitation, 30* (4), 579–590.

McNett, M., Sarver, W. and Wilczewski, P. (2012). The prevalence, treatment and outcomes of agitation among patients with brain injury admitted to acute care units. *Brain Injury, 26*, 1155–1162. https://doi.org/10.3109/02699052.2012.667587

Mental Health Act (2007). London: Her Majesty's Stationery Office.

Mortimer, D.S. and Berg, W. (2017). Agitation in patients recovering from traumatic brain injury: Nursing management. *Journal of Neuroscience Nursing, 49* (1), 25–30.

Mortimer, D., Trevena-Peters, J., McKay, A. and Ponsford, J. (2019). Economic evaluation of activities of daily living retraining during posttraumatic amnesia for inpatient rehabilitation following severe traumatic brain injury. *Archives of Physical Medicine and Rehabilitation, 100* (4), 648–655. https://doi.org/10.1016/j.apmr.2018.08.184

Nash, R.P., Weinberg, M.S., Laughon, S.L., McCall, R.C., Bateman, J.R. and Rosenstein, D.L. (2019). Acute pharmacological management of behavioral and emotional dysregulation following a traumatic brain injury: A systematic review of the literature. *Psychosomatics, 60* (2), 139–152.

Nott, M.T., Chapparo, C. and Baguley, I.J. (2006). Agitation following traumatic brain injury: An Australian sample, *Brain Injury, 20* (11), 1175–1182. https://doi.org/10.1080/02699050601049114

Pelser, C., Banks, H. and Bavikatte, G. (2023). *A Practical Approach to Interdisciplinary Complex Rehabilitation*. London: Elsevier.

Ponsford, J.L., Spitz, G. and McKenzie, D. (2016). Using post-traumatic amnesia to predict outcome after traumatic brain injury. *Journal of Neurotrauma, 33* (11), 997–1004. https://doi.org/10.1089/neu.2015.4025

Scottish Intercollegiate Guidelines Network (SIGN) (2013). *Brain Injury Rehabilitation in Adults*. Edinburgh: SIGN. Available from: https://www.sign.ac.uk/media/1068/sign130.pdf

Smart, E. and Teager, A. (2018). Exploring the acceptability and feasibility of developing a reflective practice group on an acute inpatient neurorehabilitation ward. Presented at *University of Manchester Doctorate in Clinical Psychology (DClinPsy) Annual Review*, Manchester, UK.

Soreny, C. (2009). Neuroscience nurses' perceptions of caring for challenging patients. *British Journal of Neuroscience Nursing, 5* (9), 425–431. https://doi.org/10.12968/bjnn.2009.5.9.44100

Steel, J., Ferguson, A., Spencer, E. and Togher, L. (2015). Language and cognitive communication during post-traumatic amnesia: A critical synthesis. *NeuroRehabilitation, 37* (2), 221–234.

Steel, J., Ferguson, A., Spencer, E. and Togher, L. (2017). Language and cognitive communication disorder during post-traumatic amnesia: Profiles of recovery after TBI from three cases. *Brain Injury, 31* (13–14), 1889–1902.

Tate, R.L., Pfaff, A., Baguley, I.J., Marosszeky, J.E., Gurka, J.A., Hodgkinson, A.E. and Hanna, J. (2006). A multicentre, randomised trial examining the effect of test procedures measuring emergence from post-traumatic amnesia. *Journal of Neurology, Neurosurgery and Psychiatry, 77* (7), 841–849.

Thomas, D. (2009). The journey back to effective cognitive function after brain injury. A patient perspective. *International Journal of Therapy and Rehabilitation, 16* (9), 497–501.

Thomas, H., Feyz, M., LeBlanc, J., Brosseau, J., Champoux, M.C., Christopher, A., Desormeaux, N., Dorais, L. and Lin, H. (2003). North Star Project: Reality orientation in an acute care setting for patients with traumatic brain injuries. *The Journal of Head Trauma Rehabilitation, 18* (3), 292–302.

Trevena-Peters, J., McKay, A. and Ponsford, J. (2017). *Therapy Manual: Retraining Activities of Daily Living During Post-Traumatic Amnesia following Traumatic Brain Injury*. Sydney, Australia: ASSBI Resources.

Trevena-Peters, J., McKay, A. and Ponsford, J. (2019). Activities of daily living retraining and goal attainment during posttraumatic amnesia. *Neuropsychological Rehabilitation, 29* (10), 1655–1670. https://doi.org/10.1080/09602011.2018.1441033

Trevena-Peters, J., Ponsford, J. and McKay, A. (2018). Agitated behavior and activities of daily living retraining during posttraumatic amnesia. *The Journal of Head Trauma Rehabilitation, 33* (5), 317–325.

Watts, K., and Teager, A.J. (2022, November 7). Retrospective analysis of referrals for neuropsychology input in a hyper-acute neurorehabilitation service [Poster presentation]. *United Kingdom Acquired Brain Injury Time for Change Summit*, Manchester, UK. http://dx.doi.org/10.13140/RG.2.2.21398.63040

Weir, N., Doig, E.J., Fleming, J.M., Wiemers, A. and Zemljic, C. (2006). Objective and behavioural assessment of the emergence from post-traumatic amnesia (PTA). *Brain Injury, 20* (9), 927–935.

Yuen, H.K. and Benzing, P. (1996). Guiding of behaviour through redirection. *Brain Injury Rehabilitation, 10* (3), 229–238.

11 The clinical realities of delivering neurobehavioural rehabilitation in the community

Jenny Brooks and Clark Gilkes

Introduction

NbR was pioneered in the UK at the Kemsley Unit, St Andrews Hospital, Northampton, which began admitting patients in 1979. Eames and Wood (1985) reported on the first cohort of 24 patients with ABI who participated in this unique rehabilitation programme. Since this early work, NbR has continued to evolve as a discipline and a robust evidence base supporting its use has been established (Wood, Alderman and Worthington, 2020). NbR has been demonstrated to be a cost-effective and clinically effective rehabilitation approach (Alderman, Knight and Brooks, 2013; Alderman and Wood, 2013; Oddy and da Silva Ramos, 2013; Wood et al., 1999). Individuals referred to NbR services are typically excluded, or do not benefit from, traditional neurorehabilitation because of neurobehavioural disability, most notably severe challenging behaviour. This can include aggression, sexually disinhibited behaviour, non-compliance or difficulties with motivation and drive (see Chapter 1).

NbR draws from several theoretical frameworks, including new learning theory, especially methods from operant conditioning, whose goals include increasing desirable behaviours and/or decreasing challenging behaviours. Due to the prevalence of neurocognitive impairment after ABI, application of these methods is necessarily informed by neuropsychological assessment. This ensures interventions are designed to take into account and circumvent neurocognitive deficits that both impair new learning and drive challenging behaviour. NbR services are organised to minimise the disabling effects of neurocognitive impairment while facilitating new learning within a positive social climate that enables fostering of therapeutic relationships (see Chapters 6 and 8).

NbR is delivered by a transdisciplinary team. Within TDT working, the pursuit and attainment of rehabilitation goals and interventions are the shared responsibility of the team and therapeutic roles are blurred. A principal advantage of this type of working is that all team members are responsible for the delivery of many aspects of rehabilitation, not just those tasks traditionally associated with their role or discipline, resulting in increased opportunities for

DOI: 10.4324/9781003083290-14

learning, as rehabilitation is not session bound. Instead, behaviour and skills are practised in real social contexts, whenever they are required.

Community neurobehavioural rehabilitation

Since the early of work of Eames and Wood (1985), research on the clinical efficacy of NbR has principally been undertaken within hospital and residential settings. NbR has also evolved a set of characteristics that clearly differentiate it from other forms of neurorehabilitation (see Chapter 8). Consequently, in the experience of the authors, these factors have resulted in a belief among some practitioners that NbR cannot be delivered within community contexts, including an individual's own home. For example, whilst one of the characteristics of NbR is that it is community facing, in that rehabilitation is extended to the community as soon as possible, a paradoxical belief held by some is that this can only be delivered when a person has been admitted into a programme based in a hospital or other residential setting. Despite this, symptoms of neurobehavioural disability are evident among many people living with the long-term consequences of ABI in community settings, including challenging behaviour (see, for example: Alderman, Williams and Wood, 2020; Tam et al., 2015; Sabaz et al., 2014). In their study, Kelly et al. (2008) found the most frequent behaviours that characterised community-dwelling adults with ABI referred for rehabilitation were verbal aggression, inappropriate social behaviours and lack of initiation (Kelly et al., 2008).

Approaches to providing behaviour support to people with various clinical conditions presenting with challenging behaviours in community settings are described in the literature. The most widely known contemporary approach is 'positive behaviour support'. PBS was originally developed to meet the needs of people with neurodevelopmental disorders. Gould et al. (2021) introduced PBS+PLUS, which was reported to be a flexible PBS intervention, utilising a person-driven collaborative approach with the aims of supporting individuals with ABI to build a meaningful life and self-regulate their behaviour. They described three cases in which PBS+PLUS was delivered to people with ABI and their carers over 12 months by a transdisciplinary team. Ponsford et al. (2022) went on to compare a group of individuals with ABI in receipt of PBS+PLUS to a compatible group on a treatment waiting list over a 12-month period. PBS+PLUS was not found to be more effective in reducing challenging behaviour than was evident in the no-treatment control group. However, a benefit was improved confidence of close others in addressing challenging behaviour in the PBS+PLUS group. Please see Chapter 8 regarding differences between NbR and PBS.

Despite the significant evidence base underpinning NbR, there are remarkably few accounts of the success of this approach when undertaken within community-based rehabilitation. In spite of this, there are reports of the cost effectiveness and clinical effectiveness of providing intensive behavioural support for individuals with ABI in community settings (for example, see Feeney et al., 2001). Furthermore, it is widely accepted in the medico-legal industry that NbR can be delivered effectively in community settings, and that independent teams, instructed via case management, are capable of reducing neurobehavioural disability and improving client outcomes.

There are many challenges to ensuring consistent delivery of NbR while working with individuals within the community and there is limited literature concerning this subject that clinicians can draw from. In the experience of the authors, chief among these challenges are: the ongoing cost of delivering neurobehavioural rehabilitation; the application of legal frameworks; management of risk; working within a TDT model; and ethical concerns about the application of behavioural methods. The clinical challenges and opportunities associated with each of these factors will be explored in the remainder of this chapter.

Challenges and opportunities in community neurobehavioural rehabilitation

Cost implications

NbR in hospital and residential settings organised specifically to support this model of care require a comprehensive clinical team, together with high levels of supervision and oversight, to ensure associated risks can be safely managed (see Chapter 4). Ideally, clinical psychologists and neuropsychologists who have experience, knowledge and specialist training regarding NbR, application of new learning theory and in the assessment and management of neurocognitive disorders, are best placed to undertake these functions. However, the availability of psychologists in any context is limited and can be expensive. In practice, a wider team will be required to facilitate neurorehabilitation in a community context and the expense of the psychologist will form a portion of a wider package of costs required to secure input from other rehabilitation disciplines. This creates more challenges for funding. Professionals involved with securing funds (e.g., case managers, care coordinators) can utilise the research literature, which provides a robust evidence base of NbR being both cost effective and clinically effective in the longer term (Oddy and da Silva Ramos, 2013).

A further consideration regarding costs is that NbR is not a 'quick fix' and funds need to be secured to ensure gains made in rehabilitation can be maintained over time. Availability and use of appropriate clinical measurement and outcome measures can be used to demonstrate the level of risk and clinical needs, as well as progress over time and the impact of current levels of supervision and input. Within NbR, assessing clinical needs, formulation, designing behaviour support plans and monitoring progress, are underpinned through use of instruments specifically conceptualised for use in neurorehabilitation. One such instrument is the 'St Andrews–Swansea Neurobehavioural Outcome Scale' (Alderman, Wood and Williams, 2011), which enables detailed analysis of symptoms of neurobehavioural disability; the repeated administration of the SASNOS allows these to be monitored over time. A particular advantage of the SASNOS is the availability of optional dependency ratings that assessors complete for each item that reflect the level of supervision and input the person is receiving. This enables item weighting to reflect an individual's levels of autonomy and support given within the context that the assessment is made (Alderman, Williams and Wood, 2017). Whilst ratings may suggest symptoms of neurobehavioural disability fall within the range expected in the general population, this may be attributable to the level of support the person is in receipt of. When the context is a rehabilitation unit, high levels of structure and support may suppress behaviour and other symptoms that would otherwise be present. Weighting scores according to the level of support received can be invaluable in demonstrating what might happen should the person move to another context in which this support is not available. See Figure 11.1 for an example of this. Other measures include the 'Overt Aggression Scale – Modified for Neurorehabilitation' (Alderman, Knight and Morgan, 1997) and the 'St Andrews Sexual Behaviour Assessment' (Knight, Alderman, Johnson, Green, Birkett-Swan and Yorstan, 2008), which have both been specifically designed for use in NbR. They enable the collection of detailed information from direct observation of behaviour, and this has many uses, including assessment and functional analysis as well as demonstrating clinical need, progress over time and the clinical efficacy of individual behaviour support plans (see Chapter 5). As they have been conceptualised for NbR, the use of these measures carries some authority regarding a justification for staffing levels and costs.

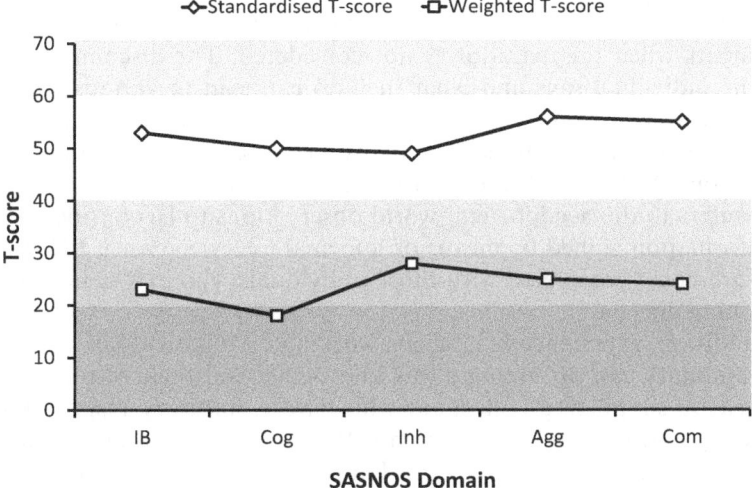

Figure 11.1 Comparison of standardised and weighted T-scores from the SAS-NOS. Whilst standardised scores all fall in what is considered the normal range for neurologically healthy people (40–60), scores that are weighted to reflect the level of support given within that context suggest that, if this was withdrawn, significant symptoms of neurobehavioural disability would return.

Legal challenges

Ensuring the individual's care and treatment is supported by the correct legal framework is imperative to the delivery of rehabilitation (see Chapter 3).

In the UK, within community settings, the Mental Capacity Act (2005) is the predominant legal framework utilised. Individuals with ABI may lack capacity in making some decisions (for example, with regard to their care and treatment) because of neurocognitive impairments. The MCA outlines that the individual being assessed has to have a disturbance or impairment in their brain or mind and that this relates to the point in time when a decision needs to be made. The MCA further demands that the individual needs to be able to understand relevant information, use and weigh up this information, retain the information long enough to make a decision, and communicate this.

Impairment of executive functions are also a frequent outcome of ABI. Executive functioning is an umbrella term for set of cognitive processes typically associated with prefrontal brain structures, including working memory, planning, problem solving, flexibility, self-monitoring and inhibitory control. This can result in an individual being unable to translate intention into action, whilst appearing seemingly plausible. Some people with frontal lobe damage can perform well in interview and test settings, despite marked difficulties in everyday life, as a result of executive functioning impairment. This is known as the 'frontal lobe paradox', consequences of which are cognitive and behaviour challenges that negatively impact on the individual's ability to be capacitous.

George and Gilbert (2018) highlighted the ongoing challenges of MCA assessments when this paradox is not considered. The disconnect between what the individual says and what they do can lead to various risks being overlooked when MCA assessments are conducted using solely a structured interview, especially when assessors have no experience or training in outcomes from ABI. The National Institute for Clinical Excellence (NICE) (2018) refers to the need for real-world observations to be considered alongside information gained by means of a formal interview, when MCA assessments are being completed with those individuals who experience executive functioning deficits.

In addition, experienced clinicians working with individuals with ABI in the community can disseminate this knowledge and their own expertise in this area by supporting colleagues who have a statutory responsibility to complete particular MCA assessments. Working in unison and asking curious questions is the ideal approach. Examples of this could include having two assessors completing MCA assessments (e.g., a brain injury expert, supporting those with statutory responsibility), assessors fact-checking information from interviews with clients with other professionals or family members, and assessors reviewing clinical documents for evidence of real-world functioning.

Challenges regarding risk management

Managing risk within the community comes with many challenges. Examples include disagreement about an individual's capacity to consent to care and treatment that may raise concerns (e.g., an individual refusing treatment and/ or supervision designed to reduce or mitigate risk). Another example is, in contrast to the specialised environments of NbR services, in the community there is reduced ability to use environmental factors as part of a risk management plan. Finally, staff burnout and turnover are risk factors to the ongoing sustainability of a community rehabilitation package.

Clinicians can address capacity concerns through ensuring good practice guidelines are adhered to – for example, with regard to the frontal lobe paradox discussed above. In addition, use of observational recordings measures, including the OAS-MNR and SASBA, which provide accessible and detailed information, can support risk assessment and ensure regular review of such documents are data-driven and evidence-based. Identification of a defined threshold for risk will inform risk and safety planning as well as behavioural contracting.

Community settings are typically perceived to be less predictable than specialised inpatient services, with the perception that there are fewer options available to use the environment to manage risk. This often becomes a significant and understandable concern for clinicians discharging individuals from inpatient or residential units into the community. The role of the environment in NbR is to help minimise the effects of neurocognitive impairment and facilitate new learning. However, within community settings, environments can be adapted to reduce demands on cognitive vulnerabilities, often in a more individualised way, than is possible in an inpatient or residential unit. This can include the use of signage, audio and visual reminders, alarms, timetables and calendars. Such specific and detailed individualisation of an environment can contribute towards risk management (e.g., reduced frustration) and set up an environment that is conducive for learning.

Behavioural disturbance after ABI can be primarily underpinned by neurocognitive disorder, most commonly executive dysfunction (e.g., Alderman, 2003). However, this can be further exacerbated by environmental factors. A common function of challenging behaviour after ABI is to serve an escape/ avoidance function (Alderman, 2001) and the stressors associated with shared living may negatively impact behaviour (Pryor, 2004). Within community living, environmental factors associated with behavioural disturbance can be reduced. This can include setting events, such as noise, and the absence of antecedents, such as behavioural disturbance in fellow patients/residents that may or may not be directed at the individual.

The importance of choice in healthcare has been highlighted in various government mandates, with individuals with long-term conditions specifically highlighted. Choice may be restricted in part in inpatient and residential units due to the nature of group and/or institutionalised living. There is the potential for choice to be less restricted within community rehabilitation packages through bespoke design, with the individual, where their choices and wishes can be utilised, whenever it is safe to do so. This may include environmental factors such as the type of bed and mattress a person can choose to sleep on, to decoration preferences, or the timing of meals, when contact can be had with family and friends and, to some extent, how daily activities are planned. Furthermore, the person with brain injury can be involved in the interviewing of support staff. For those with open litigation cases, independent advocacy can be funded through their claim.

Staff challenges including TDT working

An important part of risk planning is a rolling training programme for staff. Such training can support understanding of the clinical application of the NbR model and ensure that plans to manage risk behaviours are evidence-based.

It is well recognised that healthcare professionals are vulnerable to experiencing stress, compassion fatigue and secondary trauma. Reflective practice groups have been found to assist in mitigating these risks. Within such groups, a structured approach is taken to provide space for staff to think about the complexity of the clinical situations they work within and how this can be emotionally charged (Kurtz, 2019). Kurtz makes the link between developments within the neuroscience literature and reflective practice, and further highlights the work of van der Kolk (2014), which shows how heightened stress activates parts of the mind and body involved in defensive action, and deactivates those that generate creative and relational thinking. Kurtz (2019) argues both the importance (and difficulty) for healthcare staff to transition within reflective practice groups from a stressed, emotionally charged state to a more reflective and analytical one. Therefore, the provision of reflective practice groups within community NbR is an important consideration, especially when some workers may work predominantly in isolation (e.g., support workers).

As discussed earlier and elsewhere in this volume (for example, see Chapter 8), working as a TDT is a key component of NbR. This necessitates a blurring of clinical roles, meaning clinicians may be working outside of the traditional tasks typically associated with their discipline or role. This may be an unfamiliar way of working to many, compared to the usual clinical approach of specific disciplines holding specific responsibilities and completing certain duties and tasks. Formal training, role-modelling, supervision and use of outcome measures to demonstrate the necessary investment in this model are all imperative.

Within inpatient or residential units, the typical set up of the clinical teams and the shared work environment provides regular discussions (both structured and impromptu) about clients, facilitating regular review and decision-making opportunities. This is a potential vulnerability within community settings, where opportunities for such reviews are reduced, threatening the ability to make timely decisions in response to risk and presenting clinical needs. However, the creative application of technology can go some way to reduce this challenge. Employing shared drives to store documents and protect their content, group messaging applications, teleconferencing, and scheduling regular reviews can be considered. These can support the ability of community teams to ensure consistent and reliable methods of communication, while maintaining data security and data protection. Furthermore, storage and availability of risk and crisis management plans can ensure that teams know how to respond should issues arise. It is important to instruct a key individual (e.g., case manager) to oversee team communication and cohesion and ensure there is consistent dissemination of key information as well as coordinate and lead team clinical reviews.

Challenges for choice of interventions

As previously discussed, including in Chapters 2 and 4 of this volume, making a decision to intervene in an attempt to change an individual's behaviour will inevitably raise ethical and moral questions. These questions may be harder to answer in community settings, where, for example, the person is living in their own home. As with any other intervention being delivered as part of a community rehabilitation programme, safeguards should be maintained for the individual by an appropriate legal framework. In the UK, an MCA assessment should be completed if there are queries about an individual's capacity to consent. The design and review of behavioural interventions should be evidence-based and driven by objective data. Use of appropriate measurement instruments, such as the OAS-MNR and SASBA, will support ongoing functional analysis and allow the review of the efficacy of specific interventions.

The involvement of the individual and relevant others (e.g., family, or TDT members) is another important factor in the design and review of such interventions and contributes to the sustainability of behaviour support plans over time. As previously described, assessment of an individual's neurocognitive profile should also be considered, both in determining the extent to which it maintains behaviour and in the design of the intervention. As mentioned throughout this volume, new learning theories, including operant learning, are key concepts, and the use of methods utilising positive reinforcement are optimal in not only specialised NbR services but also community rehabilitation. Reinforcement may take many forms, depending on what is relevant and reinforcing for that individual. As within any setting, agreement with the individual and relevant others, or through the best interest process for those individuals who lack capacity, is key to ensuring that agreed reinforcement is delivered. Tangible reinforcers within a community context may include 'therapeutic earnings' (i.e., being paid a 'wage' to engage in aspects of rehabilitation or, perhaps, in additional leisure activities).

Case example

Having described typical challenges to undertaking NbR in community settings, a fictional case study will now be described to illustrate how some of these are able to be resolved.

Pauline, a 45-year-old woman, sustained a traumatic brain injury as a result of a road traffic accident ten years previously. Prior to injury, Pauline completed higher education, receiving a BSc in Criminology. She went on to work as a legal secretary.

NbR in a specialised service

Following her acute treatment in a major trauma centre, Pauline was admitted into an NbR service because of ongoing incidents of aggression. Due to the level of risk she posed to others, she was legally detained under the Mental Health Act. Neurocognitive testing indicated that Pauline's IQ was in the low average range, which was a marked decline compared with pre-morbid predictions on formal tests. She also had cognitive and behaviour vulnerabilities in aspects of executive functioning, including working memory, insight, self-monitoring, poor motivation and regulation of her emotion and behaviour. Pauline scored highly on a measure of fatigue. Functional assessment of Pauline's aggressive behaviour was undertaken using observational data collected using the OAS-MNR. It was found that she engaged in verbal and physical aggression towards others, typically in response to members of the rehabilitation team prompting her to engage in daily tasks, such as washing, dressing, and attending meals and scheduled rehabilitation sessions. As a consequence, she spent a lot of her day in bed. When her behaviour and limited engagement were discussed with her, Pauline denied there was an issue and often became agitated. It was formulated that Pauline's aggressive behaviour and lack of engagement in daily living tasks and her rehabilitation were secondary to deficits in executive functioning, specifically difficulties with working memory, insight, self-monitoring, poor motivation and regulation of her emotion and behaviour, further exacerbated by high levels of fatigue. The OAS-MNR recordings demonstrated a build-up in aggression, with Pauline often initially engaging in personal insults and direct threats of aggression, which then could escalate to physical assaults on staff, at times causing minor injury.

A behaviour support plan was created by the team, led by the consultant clinical neuropsychologist. This made reference to structured, timetabled rehabilitation sessions, aimed at increasing Pauline's insight into her needs and supporting her psychosocial adjustment. Furthermore, a sleep hygiene plan and scheduled daytime naps were introduced into Pauline's timetable. A positive reinforcement programme with social and tangible reinforcers to increase the likelihood of Pauline completing daily activities and attending sessions was put in place, with expectations increasing in line with her progress.

In addition, a response-cost programme was designed with Pauline to target her aggression, and the staff team received specific training on how to deliver it. Monitoring on the OAS-MNR revealed that, over time, the frequency and severity of aggression reduced. The OAS-MNR recordings demonstrated the efficacy of this programme in reducing verbal aggression and preventing the escalation of physical aggression towards others. Attempts to withdraw the response-cost programme were unsuccessful, with Pauline's behaviour escalating in both frequency and severity. As a result, this programme was maintained.

Pauline was subsequently discharged from section under the Mental Health Act, but due to her lack of capacity to consent to her care and treatment and residency, a Deprivation of Liberty Safeguards was put in place. Due to Pauline's continued progress, she was deemed suitable to be discharged into the community. It was recognised that her behavioural programmes had proved to be instrumental in the reduction of her aggressive behaviour and engagement and therefore needed to be maintained in the community.

Challenges to continuing NbR in the community

Legal challenges

A reassessment of Pauline's capacity to consent to care and treatment was completed by the community TDT and she was found to continue to lack capacity in this area. The inpatient TDT and community TDT worked together to draft a risk assessment and care plan. Both teams, along with statutory services, Pauline and her family, attended the best interest meeting. Following this meeting and, as outlined in Chapter 3, an application was made to the Court of Protection (a superior court having jurisdiction over property, financial affairs and personal welfare for those individuals deemed to lack capacity to make such decisions) with the order being in place on discharge.

At times, other professionals and agencies became involved in Pauline's care and questioned her capacity to consent to her care and treatment, due to her levels of plausibility in the moment. Information on the frontal lobe paradox (a disconnect between what she would say and what she would do) was shared at these times to ensure requests for and/or repeat capacity assessments were carried out as per recommendations for people experiencing difficulties secondary to executive function impairment.

Challenges regarding choice of interventions

A consultant clinical neuropsychologist was appointed to lead Pauline's community NbR programme. A support team was recruited and members received training on ABI and NbR (which included the use of the OAS-MNR and delivery of Pauline's behavioural programmes). Pauline reported to enjoy living within her own home, and engaged in many activities within her community, such as joining the gym, being part of a walking club and spending time in her local coffee shop. Pauline often had times when her behaviour increased and/or she started to disengage in daily tasks. At these times, members of the TDT would question the ongoing NbR programme and its ability to manage Pauline's ongoing behavioural needs. Such issues were discussed in reflective practice sessions, helping staff to consider what may have influenced the increase in behavioural disturbance and/or changes in her levels of engagement. Such reflections led to Pauline's timetable being reviewed, her behavioural programmes having amendments made and initiatives to ensure consistency of the delivery of her rehabilitation programme.

Challenges regarding risk management

Pauline's risk assessment and risk management plan was created and regularly reviewed by all members of the TDT. Engagement with local services took place prior to discharge to discuss crisis management planning. The agreement regarding what would trigger a referral to such services was documented in a crisis risk management plan and discussed with Pauline.

Staff challenges – TDT working

The case manager coordinating Pauline's care and treatment held responsibility for ensuring the team were working within a TDT model. The case manager ensured the team had identified shared goals with Pauline and that these were reflected in the care plans and update reports. Furthermore, an online secure platform was in place for team members to share relevant documents. Regular clinical reviews were scheduled. Team members were encouraged to work with Pauline alongside support workers (rather than in a separate room) so role-modelling and handover of rehabilitation strategies and programmes could take place.

Cost implications

Ongoing funding for Pauline's care package was regularly questioned, given that the data showed a reduction or, at times, absence of challenging behaviour. In response to this, the sharing of behavioural data over time demonstrated the impact of the behavioural programme in place, as well regular spikes in behavioural recordings and the need for expert review and changes to her programme.

Summary and conclusions

NbR has a robust evidence base that confirms it is both a clinical- and cost-effective intervention for individuals with acquired brain injury who present with severe symptoms of neurobehavioural disability, including challenging behaviour. The literature reflects that NbR has typically been delivered in inpatient and residential units, with a limited focus regarding its application to community contexts. This has led to a misperception among some clinicians that NbR cannot be delivered within the community.

The practical delivery of community NbR has its challenges, such as ongoing costs, the use of legal frameworks, managing risk and ensuring consistent delivery of targeted interventions through transdisciplinary working. However, as has been illustrated in this chapter, these challenges can be mitigated through: reference to the evidence base; brain injury specialists leading the rehabilitation programme and informing and supporting the legal frameworks process; recognising the role of the environment in managing risk as well as promoting learning and fostering therapeutic relationships; training of staff; fostering reflective practice; and ensuring excellent coordination of resources and communication supported by the advances in technology.

References

Alderman, N. (2001). Management of challenging behaviour. In Wood, R.Ll. and McMillan, T. (eds), *Neurobehavioural Disability and Social Handicap Following Traumatic Brain Injury*. Hove: Psychology Press.

Alderman, N. (2003). Contemporary approaches to the management of irritability and aggression following traumatic brain injury. *Neuropsychological Rehabilitation, 13* (1–2), 211–240.

Alderman, N., Knight, C. and Brooks, J. (2013). Rehabilitation approaches to the management of aggressive behaviour disorders after acquired brain injury. *Brain Impairment, 14* (10), 5–20.

Alderman, N., Knight, C. and Morgan, C. (1997). Use of a modified version of the Overt Aggression Scale in the measurement and assessment of aggressive behaviours following brain injury. *Brain Injury, 11* (7), 503–523.

Alderman, N., Williams, C. and Wood, R.Ll. (2017). When normal scores don't equate to independence: Recalibrating ratings of neurobehavioural disability from the 'St Andrew's–Swansea Neurobehavioural Outcome Scale' to reflect context-dependent support. *Brain Injury, 32* (2), 218–229.

Alderman, N., Williams, C. and Wood, R.Ll. (2020). Using the St Andrew's–Swansea Neurobehavioural Outcome Scale (SASNOS) to determine prevalence and predictors of neurobehavioural disability amongst survivors with traumatic brain injury in the community. *Neuropsychological Rehabilitation, 32* (1), 1–28.

Alderman, N. and Wood, R.Ll. (2013). Neurobehavioural approaches to the rehabilitation of challenging behaviour. *Neurorehabilitation, 32* (4), 761–770.

Alderman, N., Wood, R.Ll. and Williams, C. (2011). The development of the St Andrew's–Swansea Neurobehavioural Outcome Scale: Validity and reliability of a new measure of neurobehavioural disability and social handicap. *Brain Injury, 25* (1), 83–100.

Eames, P. and Wood, R.Ll. (1985). Rehabilitation after severe brain injury: A follow up study of a behaviour modification approach. *Journal of Neurology, Neurosurgery, and Psychiatry, 48* (7), 613–619.

Feeney, T.J., Ylvisaker, M., Rosen, B.H. and Greene, P (2001). Community supports for individuals with challenging behavior after brain injury: An analysis of the New York State Behavioral Resource Project. *Journal of Head Trauma Rehabilitation, 16* (1), 61–75.

George, M. and Gilbert, S. (2018). Mental Capacity Act (2005) assessments: Why everyone needs to know about the frontal lobe paradox. *The Neuropsychologist, 5*, 59–66.

Gould, K.R., Ponsford, J.L., Hicks, A.J., Hopwood, M., Renison, B. and Feeney, T.J. (2021). Positive behaviour support for challenging behaviour after acquired brain injury: An introduction to PBS+PLUS and three case studies. *Neuropsychological Rehabilitation, 31* (1), 57–59.

Kelly, G., Brown, S., Todd, J. and Kremer, P. (2008). Challenging behaviour profiles of people with acquired brain injury living in community settings. *Brain Injury, 22* (6), 457–470.

Knight, C., Alderman, N., Johnson, C., Green, S., Birkett-Swan, L. and Yorstan, G. (2008). The St Andrew's Sexual Behaviour Assessment (SASBA): Development of a standardised recording instrument for the measurement and assessment of challenging sexual behaviour in people with progressive and acquired neurological impairment. *Neuropsychological Rehabilitation*, 8 (2), 129–159.

Kurtz, A. (2019). *How to Run Reflective Practice Groups*. Abingdon: Routledge.

Mental Capacity Act (2005). London: HMSO.

National Institute for Health and Care Excellence (NICE) (2018) Decision-making and mental capacity NICE guideline [NG108] Available at: https://www.nice.org.uk/guidance/ng108/chapter /Recommendations#assessment-of-mental-capacity.

Oddy, M. and da Silva Ramos, S. (2013). The clinical and cost-benefits of investing in neurobehavioural rehabilitation: a multi-centre study. *Brain Injury*, 27, 1500–1507.

Ponsford, J.L., Hicks, A.J., Gould, K.R., Downing, M.G., Hopwood, M. and Feeney, T.J. (2022). Positive behaviour support for adults with acquired brain injury and challenging behaviour: A randomised controlled trial. *Annals of Physical and Rehabilitation Medicine*, 65 (2), 101604.

Pryor, J. (2004). What environmental factors irritate people with acquired brain injury? *Disability and Rehabilitation*, 26 (16), 974–980.

Sabaz, M.K., Simpson, G.K., Walker, A.J., Rogers, J.M., Gillis, I. and Strettles, B. (2014). Prevalence, comorbidities, and correlates of challenging behavior among community-dwelling adults with severe traumatic brain injury: A multicenter study. *Journal of Head Trauma Rehabilitation*, 29 (2), 19–30.

Tam, S., McKay, A., Sloan, S. and Ponsford, J. (2015). The experience of challenging behaviours following severe TBI: A family perspective. *Brain Injury*, 29, 813–821.

van der Kolk. B. (2014). *The Body Keeps the Score: Mind Brain and Body in the Transformation of Trauma*. London: Penguin Books.

Wood, R.Ll., Alderman, N. and Worthington, A. (2020). Neurobehavioural rehabilitation. In N. Agrawal, R. Faruqui and M. Bodani (eds), *Oxford Textbook of Neuropsychiatry* (475–481). Oxford: Oxford University Press.

Wood, R.Ll., McCrea, J.D., Wood, L.M. and Merriman, R.N. (1999). Clinical and cost effectiveness of post-acute neurobehavioural rehabilitation. *Brain Injury*, 13 (2), 69–88.

12 Managing behaviour in functional neurological disorders

Andrew Worthington, Abigail Methley and Alistair Teager

Introduction

This chapter addresses the challenges of managing behaviour associated with functional neurological conditions. Although the topic is absent from other texts on behavioural management following acquired brain injury this is due to the prevailing distinction between organic and non-organic causes of behaviour disturbance. Such a dichotomy fails to recognise the common ground in terms of behavioural overlap, neuroscience and treatment approaches. In the present chapter we review the nature of functional neurological disorder (FND), starting with a brief historical background and an overview of key terms and concepts, and noting the wide range of functional presentations before addressing challenges in assessment, formulation and management. The key message of the present chapter is that it is important for professionals who work with people who have sustained a brain injury to remain mindful of the multitude of ways in which behaviour may mimic the features of structural brain damage and to be able to adapt their interventions accordingly to ensure appropriate formulation and effective rehabilitation.

Brief history of functional neurological disorders

The familiar term hysteria reflects classical (Greek) notions of the uterine origins of a range of otherwise unexplained behaviours and is associated with Hippocrates of Kos (c.460 BCE–c.375 BCE) and later Galen (c.130–c.210). The French physician Charles Le Pois (1563–1633) is credited with being the first to recognise the cerebral origins of hysteria. Historically there has been much debate as to whether hysteria was a psychological disorder or an illness of the nervous system (Scull, 2009), an ambiguity reflected in the term functional neurological disorder. In examination of hysterical symptoms, the frequent absence of clues to their origin led Freud to speculate about hidden (repressed) memories, famously stating that 'hysterics suffer for the most part from reminiscences' (Freud & Breuer, 1893/1908, p. 11). In fact, psychiatric disturbance is probably no more common in FND than in other neurological conditions. Freud's early mentor, Jean-Martin Charcot, by contrast spent much of his

DOI: 10.4324/9781003083290-15

career viewing hysteria through the lens of neurological disease, his work incorporating many symptoms recognisable as FND today. A century later, Szasz regarded hysteria in quasi-political terms as a game involving inequalities: 'hysteria is a form of non-verbal communication … a system of rule-following behaviour, making special use of the rules of helplessness, illness and coercion', (Szasz, 1972, p. 25). While Charcot's legacy is resurgent in contemporary notions of FND, the importance of cultural norms, beliefs and expectations is also to be found in current neuropsychological models of behaviour in FND.

Functional neurological disorders

Scientific literature is replete with references to hysteria, conversion disorder and Briquet's syndrome, somatoform disorder, dissociative disorder, non-organic conditions, psychogenic states, medically unexplained symptoms, illness behaviour and hypochondriasis. Some of these are used interchangeably, sometimes to mean very different types of disorder, and clinicians may be confused as to what constitutes a functional neurological disorder.

Trimble (1983) traced the history of the term *functional*, citing Hughlings Jackson's use of the term to describe 'morbid alterations of the normal function of nerve tissue'. More recently, Stone, Burton and Carson (2020) defined functional neurological disorders as 'conditions whose origin arises primarily from a disorder of nervous system functioning rather than clearly identifiable pathophysiological disease'. Yet the presence of structural pathology does not always explain every neurological (behavioural) feature and the absence of identifiable pathophysiology is at best a statement of current knowledge. This is now recognised in *DSM 5* diagnostic criteria: 'the reliability of determining that a somatic symptom is medically unexplained is limited and grounding a diagnosis on the absence of an explanation is problematic and reinforces mind-body dualism' (American Psychiatric Association, 2013, p. 309).

The distinction between what is 'functional' versus 'organic', whilst deeply philosophically embedded, may not be in the best interests of a more holistic approach to brain injury rehabilitation. Stone, Carson and Hallett (2016) argued that the term 'functional' – although rather vague and equally applicable to a range of nervous system disorders – is more readily accommodated within a biopsychosocial model, places greater emphasis on mechanism than aetiology, and is more consistent with treatment objectives (to improve function). It is well placed, therefore, to find a welcome within the transdisciplinary approach that underpins neurobehavioural rehabilitation.

Behaviour in functional neurological disorders

Behaviours associated with FND are as varied as the conditions themselves. Indeed, one might say the behaviours *are* the condition, although historically the role of hidden, unconscious or repressed motives has taken centre stage. As Sullivan (2016) succinctly stated, 'the behaviour surrounding the symptom is key, not the symptom itself' (p. 18). A century ago, Head (1922) argued that diagnosis of functional symptoms (specifically hysteria) should be based on not only the absence of demonstrable organic disease but also the presence of positive signs of hysteria, by which he meant non-organic or inconsistent features. Diagnostic criteria for FND in *DSM 5* dictate that there must be evidence of incompatibility between symptoms and recognised neurological or medical conditions (e.g., Hoover's sign or a normal EEG trace). This can be difficult to establish in the context of definite brain injury, but familiarity with both plausible and non-credible neuropsychological presentations is an important asset in determining behaviours that are not explicable as structural cerebral damage. This may be easier to do for cognitive symptoms under formal neuropsychological examination as the presence of performance validity test failure has been shown to correlate self-identification with illness/injury as well as with anxiety that mental effort will exacerbate cognitive symptoms, a fear that has been termed 'cogniphobia' (Henry et al., 2018).

Since the days of Charcot and Breuer, susceptibility to suggestion has been linked to the manifestation of hysterical (now functional) symptoms. Suggestibility has also been proposed as a basis for exaggerated cognitive complaints in the absence of signs of brain damage (Delis & Wetter, 2007). How brain injury affects suggestibility is unclear, but clinicians should be aware of the potential amplification of existing symptoms or emergence of new behaviours over time. Where there is a known (structural) brain injury, the responses at a neurophysiological and behavioural level will reflect adaptation to circumstance, and functional symptoms are also likely to reflect this process at multiple levels. This is not a new idea. For Riddoch (1920), it was axiomatic that 'positive symptoms cannot be attributed to a negative lesion' as he advocated 'what Hughlings Jackson taught for so long and with so little encouragement, that symptoms and signs are not produced by destroyed tissue but are the expression of the mode of activity of what is left of the living organism' (p. 16).

The clinical focus on overt behaviours reflects that it is these behavioural indicators that characterise the condition rather than any putative underlying mechanisms. This is not because causation is unimportant but because: (i) there may not be a single root cause; (ii) the aetiology may not be identifiable; (iii) causal mechanisms are speculative; (iv) knowing a cause does not automatically indicate an intervention; and (v) addressing a historical grievance may not be necessary for effective intervention.

Neuropsychology of functional neurological disorders

The role of attention in FND can be traced to Pierre Janet's prescient insights (Janet, 1920), and attentional influences on sensorimotor and cognitive processing are now thought to correspond to different and potentially dissociable neural systems. People with FND have been shown to be more susceptible to hypnotic suggestion and, by implication, to dissociation (Wieder et al., 2022).

The presence of dissociative experience in FND supports a role for the involuntary breakdown of normally integrated mental processes such as sensation, movement, memory, awareness and identity (Pick et al., 2020). Insights from functional brain imaging studies suggest a role for limbic and frontal modulation of sensorimotor information (Vuilleumier, 2005; Burke et al., 2014), but research of this nature is in its infancy and it is difficult to draw general conclusions from different paradigms.

Recently Hallett et al., (2022) presented a model of pathophysiological mechanisms that involves a breakdown in how the brain generates a sense of agency with the result that symptoms are experienced as involuntary, a defect linked to abnormal activation at the right temporo-parietal junction. In the Bayesian model proposed by Edwards et al. (2012), the brain makes sense of the world by predicting outcomes on the basis of sensory information and prior expectation and beliefs. Functional motor and sensory symptoms occur as a result of abnormal prior beliefs, modulated by attention, and leading to prediction errors. This could arise from dysfunction of neurons encoding prior beliefs that misappropriate attention, or the dysfunction of attention networks causing rigid adherence to prior beliefs. Predisposing factors may lead to abnormal illness beliefs that mediate the focus of attention, but Edwards et al. (2012) propose that in FND the oft-reported physical precipitating event is accorded excessive weight, the abnormal belief being resistant to extinction. The authors ascribe an important role in this process to the insular cortex. This is a poorly understood region involved in a range of visceral, sensory, motor and emotional processing and implicated in a variety of neurobehavioural disorders (Nagai, Kishi and Kato, 2007), so one might justifiably consider whether brain injury could act to cause or amplify the same process that would provide a basis for the association of FND and ABI.

Functional neurological disorder and brain injury

The range of functional neurological disorders is as broad as one might encounter in a general neurology textbook. Thus the excellent *Handbook of Clinical Neurology* volume on functional neurological disorders (Hallett et al., 2016) includes chapters on the following: coma, gait disorder, tics, tremor, dystonia, paralysis, seizures, urological disorders, auditory disorders, dizziness, visual loss, eye movement disorders, facial and tongue movement disorders, swallowing disorders, voice disorders, speech disorders and amnesia. FND and brain injury are not mutually exclusive, and both may represent a brain dysfunction regardless of cause. That functional symptoms can occur in the presence of organic pathology has long been recognised. While investigating the behavioural outcomes of traumatic brain injury, Weinstein (1966) reported that functional signs were apparent in 16 out of 200 adults at some stage in their recovery. In some cases, this may be because symptoms of brain pathology provide a template for functional symptoms, which may explain the observation by Roy (1977) of a particular association between hysterical convulsions and epilepsy.

Popkirov et al. (2019) reviewed 17 studies involving 1,039 adults with non-epileptic seizures, of whom 42 per cent also reported a history of (mostly mild) head injury frequency, ranging from 16 to 83 per cent across studies.

In other instances, the organic lesion is not identified at the time. Credner (1930, cited in Merskey, 1995) found 73 cases with frontal lobe lesions in a study of 260 people suffering with symptoms regarded as hysterical. In yet other cases, the functional presentation occurs alongside the neurological presentation. For example, in Slater and Glithero's (1965) follow-up of 85 people originally labelled with hysteria, 19 were considered to have organic disease with 'hysterical overlay'.

Certain forms of brain injury might predispose people to functional behaviours. Slater and Glithero (1965) supposed that brain disorder may bring about forms of behaviour such as elaboration and attention-seeking that is typically considered hysterical (functional). Learning theory teaches that insofar as more expansive behaviour or signs of distress warrant more attention (or escape-avoidance) such actions are likely to be reinforced. Eames (1992) reviewed 167 adults with severe behaviour following ABI and identified a subgroup of 54 with atypical behaviours, reminiscent of Charcot's gross hysteria, showing inconsistencies under examination and demand-avoidance (including demonstration of 'opposite effort' – responses consistently the opposite of what is required or requested). Their apparent immunity to pleasure or pain suggested a dissociative condition, possibly involving a thalamo-cortico-gating mechanism. Interestingly they did not respond well to conventional behaviour modification methods and, as these patients had very diffuse injuries (typically anoxia, hypoglycaemia and head injury with brain swelling), it was hypothesised they sustained damage to reward systems involving the basal ganglia and diencephalon.

The challenges of functional neurological disorder

The challenges associated with FND are many and varied. There is a diagnostic challenge, the diagnosis being made using positive symptoms rather than by exclusion. Although time to diagnosis for FND is improving, there is still a lengthy delay. Kerr et al. (2021) reported an average time to diagnose dissociative seizures of 8.4 years, with delay associated with greater complexity and variability of seizures, more anti-seizure and other medications, and a history of physical abuse.

The onset of symptoms in FND is variable, relating to minor pathology such as viral illness, minor to major physical trauma and psychophysiology (e.g., the physical effects of panic and physiology, such as waking up from sleep in a paralysed state in sleep paralysis or anaesthesia) (Edwards, 2016). Symptoms can occur with or without psychological stressors. Identification of FND is also confounded by clinical complexity due to the high level of co-morbidity with FND. Many people also have a recognised neurological disorder that does not fully explain their presenting symptoms (Stone et al., 2011) and other conditions including chronic pain, headache and chronic fatigue (Carson et al., 2000). Neurodevelopmental conditions may also raise the risk of FND. Clinically a high prevalence of non-epileptic seizures is seen in people with learning disabilities, although they are often excluded from epidemiological research (Rawlings et al., 2021), and a small-scale screening study identified up to 40% of an adult sample with FND met the screening threshold for further investigation of autism (Cole, Elmalem and Petrochilos, 2023).

Poor outcomes are common in FND (Gelauff et al., 2014), with no optimum way of predicting prognosis. FND causes widespread disability and impairment, with some evidence indicating higher distress than other neurological conditions, and there are similar levels of unemployment (Carson et al., 2011), with high health care costs (£11.3 million direct healthcare costs) (Healthcare Improvement Scotland, 2012). Unfortunately access to treatment is both lengthy and variable, reflecting sparse provision and scarce expertise.

Managing the behavioural manifestations of FND is also challenging. Professionals often struggle with the formulation and clinical management of symptoms caused by a different mechanism to those more commonly encountered as a result of physical nervous system damage. Consequently, staff may lack knowledge and confidence in supporting people with these clinical needs (Lehn et al., 2019) and the level of training provision in hospital and community settings varies widely.

The problem is compounded by a lack of specialist teams, meaning people may be managed across services and experience inconsistent support and discontinuities in care. Interdisciplinary or transdisciplinary working provides the integrated treatment frequently needed but often lacking; for example, emotional needs are not addressed on medical wards or psychiatric services may lack staff trained in how to respond to physical symptoms, such as not calling an ambulance for non-epileptic attacks.

Psychosocial adversity is a risk factor for both ABI and FND. A subset of people with FND may have experienced complex trauma, including both adverse childhood experiences and acute trauma. Where trauma is known, staff also need to be confident in providing trauma-informed care generally (Portman-Thompson, 2020) and in facilitating access to appropriate specialist therapies for trauma. As in ABI, people with FND may experience higher than average levels of alexithymia (Demartini et al., 2014), making it difficult to understand and communicate their emotional needs. They may have developed methods of relating interpersonally or of regulating emotions that are experienced as challenging by staff not trained in psychological support. Staff may require skills in mental health risk assessment and in providing management and intervention around coping strategies (such as substance use and self-harm). People with FND may experience strong symptoms of panic and dissociation, and so confidence in grounding techniques is needed.

FND services and treatment settings

Depending on the attribution of symptoms, behavioural treatment of FND in the context of ABI could take place in dedicated brain injury facilities, in psychiatric settings or in generic community services. In all cases, services are likely to have significant shortfalls due to lack of knowledge and expertise. The National Neurosciences Advisory Group (2023) have set out an optimum clinical pathway for adults with FND that includes Level 1 specialist rehabilitation. In the community, however, care for people presenting with acute FND symptoms is often centred on Accident and Emergency departments (Williams et al., 2022). A lower risk of subsequent attendance at these departments can be predicted by a documented FND diagnosis, referral to clinical psychology and outpatient neurology follow-up. While not all FND is associated with emotional trauma, there is no consensus as to the most appropriate setting for trauma-specific treatment in the context of FND but a trauma-informed care pathway is required from the point of referral through to discharge. This is true not only for trauma-related FND but also for people with FND who have experienced distress through the lived experience of their symptoms and iatrogenic distress through diagnostic and treatment pathways. Yet trauma-informed pathways may not be present in physical health settings and are rare in brain injury services.

General principles of treatment

Treatment of the behavioural manifestations of FND can present a major challenge to the interdisciplinary team, especially when symptoms are chronic and entrenched. Traditional management has limited unnecessary investigations, increased the acceptability of a psychological model of symptoms and offered symptomatic treatments, regardless of the aetiology (Brown, 2004). In the absence of large-scale randomised controlled trials, several disciplines have published consensus statements outlining known clinical expertise, in order to establish an evidence base for understanding FND in occupational therapy (Nicholson et al., 2020); physiotherapy (Nielsen et al., 2015); and speech and language therapy (Baker et al., 2021).

It is important for the IDT to discuss FND respectfully, validate symptoms as genuine, ensure the evidence for the diagnosis is understood by all members of the team and provide hope for improvement. A key principle of any intervention is that FND symptoms are not viewed as intentional behaviour. It can be helpful to avoid prolonged discussion of the cause of symptoms as organic vs non-organic by referring to the growing literature on neuroimaging in FND (see Perez et al., 2021 for a review). This suggests that there are changes to both the 'software' and 'hardware' within FND, albeit the mechanisms of these hardware changes remain distinct from neurological conditions with lesion damage, and it is not yet clear if structural changes are predisposing factors or consequences (Bègue et al., 2019).

No medication is recommended for FND specifically, and some medication may be ineffective (including benzodiazepines and opiates). Medications such as antidepressants and neuropathic pain relief, which target co-morbid issues, may be helpful by improving sleep and mood and in reducing pain and anxiety.

As with ABI, psychological and behavioural interventions should not be left to psychologists or psychiatrists but embraced by the wider IDT. Even where people would benefit from specific psychological or psychiatric interventions, this may not be the first step in a stepped care model of treatment (Healthcare

Improvement Scotland, 2012). Whilst some people require specialist interventions from the outset, others may benefit from lower-level interventions, starting with self-management (see Williams et al., 2011) and cognitive behavioural therapy-based (CBT-based) strategies, supported by the IDT.

The evidence base for psychological therapies in FND is complex with significant gaps. There is currently no NICE guideline outlining best practice in psychological interventions for FND. The main psychological therapies literature focuses on CBT (Goldstein et al., 2020). Broadly, a CBT model of FND assumes that symptoms are caused by the interaction of pre-existing beliefs and conceptualisations of illness with processes of classical and operant conditioning and emotional arousal (Carson, Ludwig, & Welch, 2016). After a trigger event, a cascade of processes interact in a vicious cycle. These include cognition, such as illness beliefs and appraisals, emotions and behaviour, including safety behaviours, avoidance, symptom vigilance and monitoring, in addition to physiological changes. As with ABI, the wider context of environment, relationships and practical stressors interact to maintain symptoms and disability. Treatment aims to address these maintenance factors by changing beliefs, teaching new skills to manage emotions, and changing behaviours.

The first steps in treatment will be familiar to neurobehavioural practitioners and involve symptom checklists, completing a detailed timeline of symptoms, increasing awareness of these symptoms, and developing an understanding of any triggers. Additionally, psychoeducation includes understanding how FND is identified and reviewing the medical evidence. This might include existing neurological conditions that cannot account for the behavioural presentation as well as investigations that exclude certain causes. Crucially this is presented in a factual, non-judgemental and non-stigmatising fashion.

Psychoeducation is used to explain how the nervous system works, including the fight-flight-freeze-appease response. The mind-body link is highlighted through examples, such as panic, the physiological impact of chronic stress and the effect of chronic changes in breathing (such as hyperventilating). Key to this stage of treatment are quick and effective behavioural experiments to produce the onset of symptoms and the development of skills in relaxation and deep breathing techniques to combat this over time. Uncertainty around the cause of symptoms, their treatment and the prognosis can mean that people make decisions that ultimately, and unintentionally, maintain their symptoms, e.g., restricting the use of a muscle group or exercise more generally, which can then lead to muscle-wasting and physical decompensation. Explanation is therefore key in limiting uncertainty wherever possible to prevent these behavioural changes as early as possible. Psychoeducation helps people to understand how thoughts and symptoms are related. Thought diaries can be used to identify maladaptive cognitions and thinking styles that can be challenged in terms of their helpfulness, accuracy and balance.

Next steps can include recording the impact of activity on symptoms and learning about safety behaviours. Commonly these include excessive checking, reassurance seeking, suddenly stopping activities when symptoms begin, and distraction to avoid noticing symptoms or worries. Behaviours can then be viewed as helpful (positive cycles) or negative (vicious cycles) and, for those with the cognitive capacity, people can be assisted to make better-informed choices about their behaviour. For people with brain injury who often experience fatigue, it may be necessary to provide psychoeducation on 'boom-bust' cycles and the need for pacing.

The importance of learning and reinforcement cannot be understated, as many people with FND will avoid activities or places that are felt to make symptoms worse, reducing the opportunities to find out that the most feared outcome will not occur, increasing anxiety and decreasing confidence. This decreases people's quality of life and social connectedness more broadly. Avoidance can be subtle (such as rushing through a task) or more obvious (avoiding the task altogether). Cognitive behaviour modification strategies can be deployed to enhance quality of life by increasing activity levels, introducing or reintroducing activities that bring enjoyment and a sense of achievement and mastery, and addressing problem solving and avoidant behaviours. Where difficulties are interpersonal in nature, they may require assertiveness techniques and identification of systemic responses maintaining symptoms.

Treatment in practice: Tanya – non-epileptic attack disorder (NEAD)

Background

This is a clinical case where identifying characteristics have been changed to protect confidentiality. Tanya was a 25-year-old woman who was admitted via Accident and Emergency after repeated seizures. Video telemetry, in combination with behavioural observations on the neuroscience ward, suggested that her seizures were non-epileptic and that anti-epileptic medication was not required. Tanya found a psychological explanation for her experiences dismissive and reported feeling 'fobbed off' and being told that 'it's all in her head'. Discussions about the diagnosis resulted in her becoming agitated and verbally aggressive. Staff tried to build a therapeutic relationship with Tanya, but her behaviour ranged from dependent to avoidant. When discharge was mentioned, she became upset and either intimated suicide threats or stated that she would self-discharge. The mental health liaison team were called out every time suicidal comments were reported, but concluded that there was no immediate risk of harm to herself or others. The nursing team, who were not trained in supporting her mental health needs, felt on edge and worried for both Tanya and other patients on the ward who would be observing these events.

Formulation

An individualised formulation was discussed with Tanya and shared with her team with her consent (see Figure 12.1). With regard to broader themes from the literature of patient and professional experiences of support for NEAD

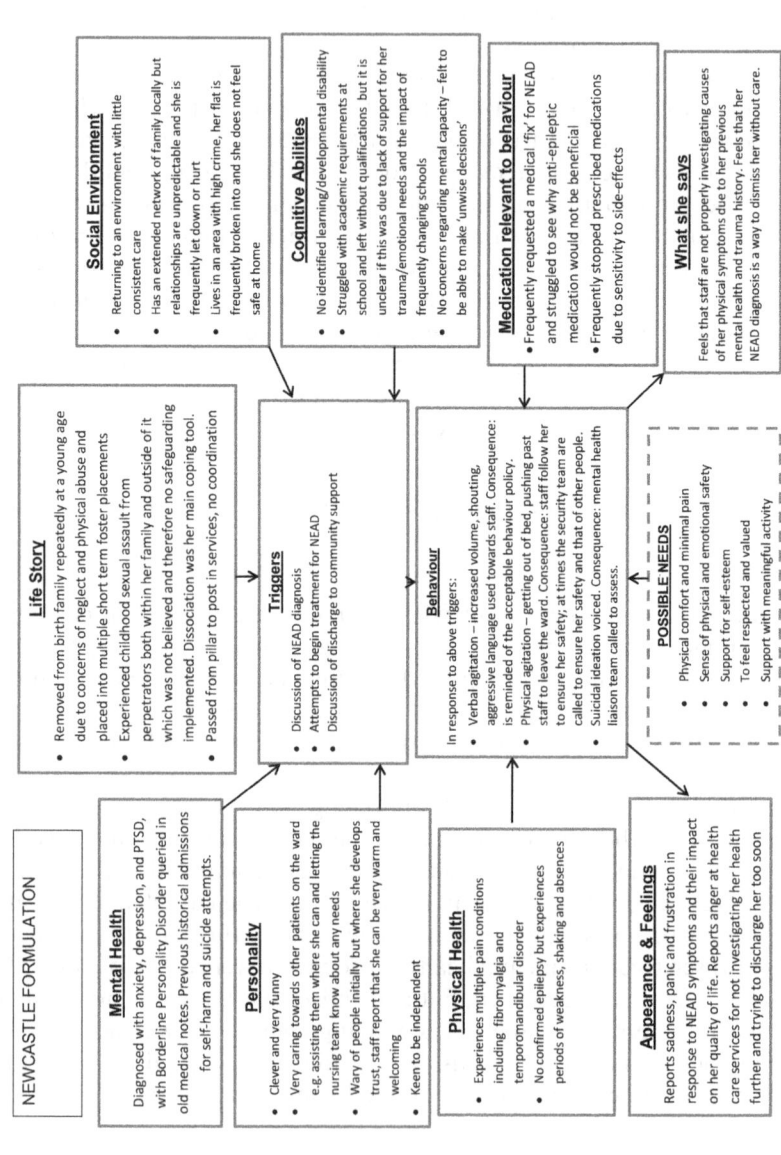

Figure 12.1 Tanya's person-centred formulation based on the biopsychosocial Newcastle model.

(Brough et al., 2015; Dickson et al. 2017), the Newcastle Model (James & Jackman, 2017) was used as a framework for formulating the difficulties the team were facing and a collaborative positive behaviour support plan developed.

Intervention

Interventions included developing a relationship and building up an understanding of Tanya's previous history, which included traumatic experiences in both her childhood and young adult years. She had not felt believed nor had she received sufficient support from formal services during these events and she was often left to cope alone. On the rare occasions where care had been provided, it was withdrawn as soon as she showed any sign of improvement, leaving her feeling abandoned and hopeless. Whilst staff did not provide therapy for these previous experiences, gaining a formulation of Tanya's experiences meant that they were able to place her engagement style within context and directly address her concerns. Using her language to describe her non-epileptic episodes showed that staff were listening to her perspective and not trying to challenge her lived experiences. Explaining her diagnosis as a 'software' and 'hardware' problem enabled her to see that her experiences were believed, respected and taken seriously. Empathising with her concerns about discharge as another abandonment enabled planning meetings with community services to provide coordination of care post-discharge. Supporting her to feel safe enough to share her feelings of hopelessness and worry, meant that suicidal comments were not needed as frequently to communicate her distress.

Team formulation sessions were used to provide staff with a private space to reflect on their experiences and process the emotions that came from supporting Tanya while she experienced these difficult and strong emotions and to provide training on active listening skills and basic emotion regulation strategies. Further training was also provided to the team on emotional and biological responses to trauma and how to deliver trauma-informed care (Portman-Thompson, 2020), as this had not been a core part of their nursing and medical training. From this, a positive behaviour support plan was created, divided into sections showing how to identify when Tanya was calm and engaged ('green'), starting to feel upset ('yellow'), very distressed ('red') and calming down after feeling distressed ('blue'). For every section accompanying strategies were listed, which helped Tanya return to the 'green' zone and stay there for as long as possible. This allowed her to accept discharge and engage more productively with support services going forward, reducing the risk of repeated cyclical hospital admissions.

Conclusion

Brain injury rehabilitation often involves working with complex clinical presentations that challenge the knowledge and skills of professionals. This is particularly the case where the nature and aetiology of behaviour is shrouded in uncertainty or contrary to expectation. FND and brain injury are not mutually exclusive, and practitioners should be aware of the potential for functional presentations within the broad spectrum of neurological conditions. Cognitive-behavioural techniques derived from learning theory and informed by cognitive neuroscience provide a sound basis for assessment and intervention as neurobehavioural rehabilitation evolves to circumvent the traditional organic/non-organic distinction and to recognise the truly neuropsychological nature of behavioural pathology.

References

American Psychiatric Association (2013). *Diagnostic and Statistical Manual of Mental Disorders Fifth Edition* (*DSM-5*). Washington, DC: American Psychiatric Publishing.

Baker, J., Barnett, C., Cavalli, L., Dietrich, M., Dixon, L., Duffy, J.R., Elias, A., Fraser, D.E., Freeburn, J.L., Gregory, C., McKenzie, K., Miller, N., Patterson, J., Roth, C., Roy, N., Short, J., Utianski, R., van Mersbergen, M., Vertigan, A., Carson, A., Stone, J. and McWhirter, L. (2021). Management of functional communication, swallowing, cough and related disorders: Consensus recommendations for speech and language therapy. *Journal of Neurology, Neurosurgery and Psychiatry*, *92* (10), 1112–1125.

Bègue, I., Adams, C., Stone, J. and Perez, D.L. (2019). Structural alterations in functional neurological disorder and related conditions: A software and hardware problem?. *NeuroImage: Clinical*, *22*, 101798.

Brough, J.L., Moghaddam, N.G., Gresswell, D.M. and Dawson, D.L. (2015). The impact of receiving a diagnosis of non-epileptic attack disorder (NEAD): A systematic review. *Journal of Psychosomatic Research*, *79* (5), 420–427.

Brown, R.J. (2004). Psychological mechanisms of medically unexplained symptoms: An integrative conceptual model. *Psychological Bulletin*, *130* (5), 793–812.

Burke, M.J., Ghaffar, O., Staines, W.R., Downar, J. and Feinstein, A. (2014). Functional neuroimaging of conversion disorder: The role of ancillary activation. *NeuroImage: Clinical*, *6*, 333–339.

Carson, A., Ludwig, L. and Welch, K. (2016). Psychologic theories in functional neurologic disorders. In M. Hallett, J. Stone and A. Carson (eds), *Handbook of Clinical Neurology* (3rd edn, Vol. 139) (pp. 105–120). Amsterdam: Elsevier.

Carson, A.J., Ringbauer, B., Stone, J., McKenzie, L., Warlow, C. and Sharpe, M. (2000). Do medically unexplained symptoms matter? A prospective cohort study of 300 new referrals to neurology outpatient clinics. *Journal of Neurology, Neurosurgery & Psychiatry*, *68* (2), 207–210.

Carson, A., Stone, J., Hibberd, C., Murray, G., Duncan, R., Coleman, R., Warlow, C., Roberts, R., Pelosi, A., Cavanagh, J., Matthews, K., Goldbeck, R., Hansen, C. and Sharpe, M. (2011). Disability, distress and unemployment in neurology outpatients with symptoms 'unexplained by organic disease'. *Journal of Neurology, Neurosurgery, and Psychiatry*, *82* (7), 810–813.

Cole, R.H., Elmalem, M.S. and Petrochilos, P. (2023). Prevalence of autistic traits in functional neurological disorder and relationship to alexithymia and psychiatric co-morbidity. *Journal of the Neurological Sciences*, *446*, 120585.

Delis, D.C. and Wetter, S.P. (2007). Cogniform disorder and cogniform condition: Proposed diagnoses for excessive cognitive symptoms. *Archives of Clinical Neuropsychology*, *22*, 589–604.

Demartini, B., Petrochilos, P., Ricciardi, L., Price, G., Edwards, M.J. and Joyce, E. (2014). The role of alexithymia in the development of functional motor symptoms (conversion disorder). *Journal of Neurology, Neurosurgery and Psychiatry*, *85* (10), 1132–1137.

Dickson, J.M., Peacock, M., Grünewald, R.A., Howlett, S., Bissell, P. and Reuber, M. (2017). Non-epileptic attack disorder: The importance of diagnosis and treatment. *BMJ Case Reports*, bcr2016218278.

Eames, P. (1992). Hysteria following brain injury. *Journal of Neurology, Neurosurgery and Psychiatry*, *55* (11), 1046–1053.

Edwards, M. (2016). Neurobiologic theories of functional neurologic disorders. In M. Hallett, J. Stone, A. Carson (eds), *Handbook of Clinical Neurology* (3rd edn; Vol. 139) (pp. 131–139). Amsterdam: Elsevier.

Edwards, M.J., Adams, R.A., Brown, H., Parees, I. and Friston, K.J. (2012). A Bayesian account of 'hysteria'. *Brain*, *135* (11), 3495–3512.

Freud, S. and Breuer, J. (1893/1908). *Studies in Hysteria*. Reprinted 2004. Harmondsworth: Penguin.

Gelauff, J., Stone, J., Edwards, M. and Carson, A. (2014). The prognosis of functional (psychogenic) motor symptoms: A systematic review. *Journal of Neurology, Neurosurgery, and Psychiatry*, *85* (2), 220–226.

Goldstein, L.H., Robinson, E.J., Mellers, J., Stone, J., Carson, A., Reuber, M., Medford, N., McCrone, P., Murray, J., Richardson, M.P., Pilecka, I., Eastwood, C., Moore, M., Mosweu, I., Perdue, I., Landau, S., Chalder, T. and CODES Study Group (2020). Cognitive behavioural therapy for adults with dissociative seizures (CODES): A pragmatic, multicentre, randomised controlled trial. *The Lancet Psychiatry*, *7* (6), 491–505.

Hallett, M. Aybek, S. Dworetzky, B.A., McWhirter, L., Staab, J.P. and Stone, J. (2022). Functional neurological disorder: New subtypes and shared mechanisms. *Lancet Neurology*, *21* (6), 537–550.

Hallett, M., Stone, J. and Carson, A. (2016). *Functional Neurologic Disorders*. Handbook of Clinical Neurology (3rd edn; Vol. 139). Amsterdam: Elsevier.

Healthcare Improvement Scotland (2012). *Stepped Care for Functional Neurological Symptoms*. Edinburgh.

Henry, G.K., Heilbronner, R.L., Suhr, J., Gornbein, J., Wagner, E., and Drane, D.L. (2018). Illness perceptions affect cognitive performance validity. *Journal of the International Neuropsychological Society*, *24*, 735–745.

James, I. A. and Jackman, L. (2017). *Understanding Behaviour in Dementia that Challenges: A Guide to Assessment and Treatment* (2nd edn). London: Jessica Kingsley.

Janet, J. (1920). *The Major Symptoms of Hysteria*. New York: Macmillan.

Kerr, W.T., Zhang, X., Hill, C.E., Janio, E.A., Chau, A.M., Braesch, C.T., Le, J.M., Hori, J.M., Patel, A.B., Allas, C.H., Karimi, A.H., Dubey, I., Sreenivasan, S.S., Gallardo, N.L., Bauirjan, J., Hwang, E.S., Davis, E.C., D'Ambrosio, S.R., Al Banna, M., Cho, A.Y., … Stern, J.M. (2021). Factors associated with delay to video-EEG in dissociative seizures. *Seizure*, *86*, 155–160.

Lehn, A., Bullock-Saxton, J., Newcombe, P., Carson, A. and Stone, J. (2019). Survey of the perceptions of health practitioners regarding functional neurological disorders in Australia. *Journal of Clinical Neuroscience*, *67*, 114–123.

Merskey, H. (1995). *The Analysis of Hysteria*. (2nd edn). London: Royal College of Psychiatrists.

Nagai, M., Kishi, K. and Kato, S. (2007). Insular cortex and neuropsychiatric disorders: A review of recent literature. *European Psychiatry*, *22* (6), 387–394.

National Neurosciences Advisory Group (2023). *Optimum Clinical Pathway for Adults: Functional Neurological Disorder.* Watford: The Neurological Alliance.

Nicholson, C., Edwards, M.J., Carson, A.J., Gardiner, P., Golder, D., Hayward, K., Humblestone, S., Jinadu, H., Lumsden, C., MacLean, J., Main, L., Macgregor, L., Nielsen, G., Oakley, L., Price, J., Ranford, J., Ranu, J., Sum, E. and Stone, J. (2020). Occupational therapy consensus recommendations for functional neurological disorder. *Journal of Neurology, Neurosurgery and Psychiatry, 91* (10), 1037–1045.

Nielsen, G., Stone, J., Matthews, A., Brown, M., Sparkes, C., Farmer, R., Masterton, L., Duncan, L., Winters, A., Daniell, L., Lumsden, C., Carson, A., David, A.S. and Edwards, M. (2015). Physiotherapy for functional motor disorders: A consensus recommendation. *Journal of Neurology, Neurosurgery and Psychiatry, 86* (10), 1113–1119.

Perez, D.L., Nicholson, T.R., Asadi-Pooya, A.A., Bègue, I., Butler, M., Carson, A.J., David, A.S., Deeley, Q., Diez, I., Edwards, M.J., Espay, A.J., Gelauff, J.M., Hallett, M., Horovitz, S.G., Jungilligens, J., Kanaan, R.A.A., Tijssen, M.A.J., Kozlowska, K., LaFaver, K., LaFrance, W.C., Jr, … Aybek, S. (2021). Neuroimaging in functional neurological disorder: State of the field and research agenda. *NeuroImage: Clinical, 30*, 102623.

Pick, S., Rojas-Aguiluz, M., Butler, M., Mulrenan, H., Nicholson, T.R. and Goldstein, L.H. (2020). Dissociation and interoception in functional neurological disorder. *Cognitive Neuropsychiatry, 25* (4), 294–311.

Popkirov, S., Asadi-Pooya, A.A., Duncan, R., Gigineishvili, D., Hingray, C., Miguel Kanner, A., LaFrance, W.C., Jr, Pretorius, C. and Reuber, M. (2019). The aetiology of psychogenic non-epileptic seizures: Risk factors and comorbidities. *Epileptic Disorders, 21* (6), 529–547.

Portman-Thompson, K. (2020). Implementing trauma-informed care in mental health services. *Mental Health Practice, 23* (3), 34–41.

Rawlings, G.H., Novakova, B., Beail, N. and Reuber, M. (2021). What do we know about non-epileptic seizures in adults with intellectual disability: A narrative review. *Seizure, 91*, 437–446.

Riddoch, G. (1920). Differential diagnosis. In: H.C. Miller (ed.), *Functional Nerve Disease* (pp. 14–17). London: Henry Frowde, Hodder & Stoughton.

Roy, A. (1977). Cerebral disease and hysteria. *Comprehensive Psychiatry, 18*, 607–609.

Scull, A (2009). *The Disturbing History of Hysteria.* New York: Oxford University Press.

Slater, E.T.O. and Glithero, E. (1965). A follow-up of patients diagnosed as suffering from 'hysteria'. *Journal of Psychosomatic Research, 9* (1): 9–13.

Stone, J., Burton, C. and Carson, A. (2020). Recognising and explaining functional neurological disorder. *British Medical Journal, 371*, m3745.

Stone, J., Carson, A., Duncan, R., Roberts, R., Coleman, R., Warlow, C., Murray, G., Pelosi, A., Cavanagh, J., Matthews, K., Goldbeck, R. and Sharpe, M. (2011). Which neurological diseases are most likely to be associated with 'symptoms unexplained by organic disease'. *Journal of Neurology, 259* (1), 33–38.

Stone, J., Carson, A. and Hallett, M. (2016). Explanation as treatment for functional neurological disorders. In M. Hallett, J. Stone and A. Carson, *Functional Neurologic Disorders. Handbook of Clinical Neurology* (3rd edn; Vol. 139) (pp. 543–553). Amsterdam: Elsevier.

Sullivan, S. (2016). *It's All in Your Head.* London: Vintage.

Szasz, T. (1972). *The Myth of Mental Illness.* London: Paladin.

Trimble, M.R. (1983). *Post-traumatic Neurosis.* Chichester: John Wiley & Son.

Vuilleumier, P. (2005). Hysterical conversion and brain function. *Progress in Brain Research*, *150*, 309–329.

Weinstein, E.A. (1966). Conversion hysteria following brain injury. *Archives of Neurology*, *15* (5), 545–548.

Wieder, L., Brown, R.J., Thompson, T. and Terhune, D.B. (2022). Hypnotic suggestibility in dissociative and related disorders: A meta-analysis. *Neuroscience & Biobehavioral Reviews*, 104751.

Williams, C., Kent, C., Smith, S., Carson, A., Sharpe, A. and Cavanagh, J. (2011). *Overcoming Functional Neurological Symptoms: A Five Areas Approach*. Oxford: Routledge.

Williams, S., Southall, C., Haley, S., Ba Dhafari, T., Kemp, S., Relton, S.D., Alty, J.E., Johnson, O., Graham, C.D. and Maguire, M. (2022). To the emergency room and back again: Circular healthcare pathways for acute functional neurological disorders. *Journal of the Neurological Sciences*, *437*, 120251.

Index